5:2 Diet For Beginners

2nd Edition

9 Steps To Lose Weight & Feel Great On A Fasting Diet – Without TRYING AT ALL!

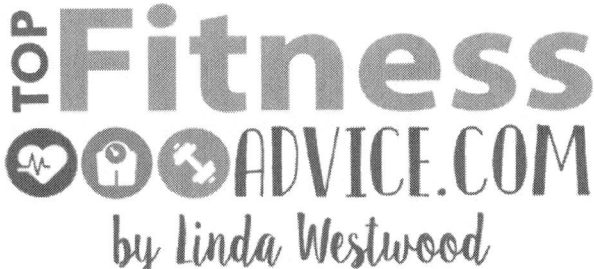

by Linda Westwood

Table Of Contents

Introduction

When you are following a strict diet plan, the most obvious problem that you encounter is what should you actually eat to remain with the diet plan diligently?

To resolve your problems, we are providing you with a few delicious recipes that you can use for your fasting days as well as for non-fasting days.

5:2 diet plan basically decides the amount of calories you are allowed to take in, on each specific day. According to this plan you will never go on a total fast day, but you will just minimize your calorie intake.

To make your each and every day worthwhile, we are giving you recipes with a total of calorie count, so that you can keep a track of calories that you have taken in one meal and thus manage rest of your day accordingly.

Chapter 1: Introduction with 5:2 Diet Plan

Let us start our book with the basic meaning of 5:2 diet plan. According to this diet plan you are supposed to fast for 2 non- consecutive days and have normal and healthy diet for 5 days.

You will need to sustain on 500 calories during these two fasting days but with the kind of diet plan and recipes we have, it is going to be very easy for you. For the rest of the 5 days, you can have 2000 calories per day. Around the world, people are widely accepting this fast diet plan and are quite happy with the output. For men, it is 600 calories and 2500 calories on 2 and 5 days respectively.

We will plan your day in such a way that you take around 100 calories in your breakfast, around 200 in your lunch and under 200 calories for your dinner. This is the way to use your 500 calories in an optimum level. We have breakfast, lunch and dinner recipes for you which will ensure good health and best taste.

Chapter 2: Functioning of 5:2 Diet Plan

5:2 diet plan is another name for intermittent fasting. Fasting is an obvious way of loosing fat because you are cutting down on your carbohydrate and fat intake. 5:2 is an efficient way in a sense that you do not go on a long term starvation mode but you follow a repair mode.

This is a diet plan which works on repairing your damaged cells so that they work in a better way. When you are on starvation mode, you are actually reinforcing your body to store more fat for future use. This method is harmful in a long term. With the help of 5:2 plan you can not only decrease the fat content of your body but also regulate the sugar level of your blood and fight diabetes in a better way.

Read This FIRST - 100% FREE BONUS

FOR A LIMITED TIME ONLY – Get Linda's best-selling book *"Quick & Easy Weight Loss: 97 Scientifically Proven Tips Even For Those With Busy Schedules!"* absolutely FREE!

Readers who have read this bonus book along with this book have seen the greatest changes in their weight loss both *FAST & EASILY* and have improved overall fitness levels – so it is *highly recommended* to get this bonus book.

Once again, as a big thank-you for downloading this book, I'd like to offer it to you *100% FREE for a LIMITED TIME ONLY!*

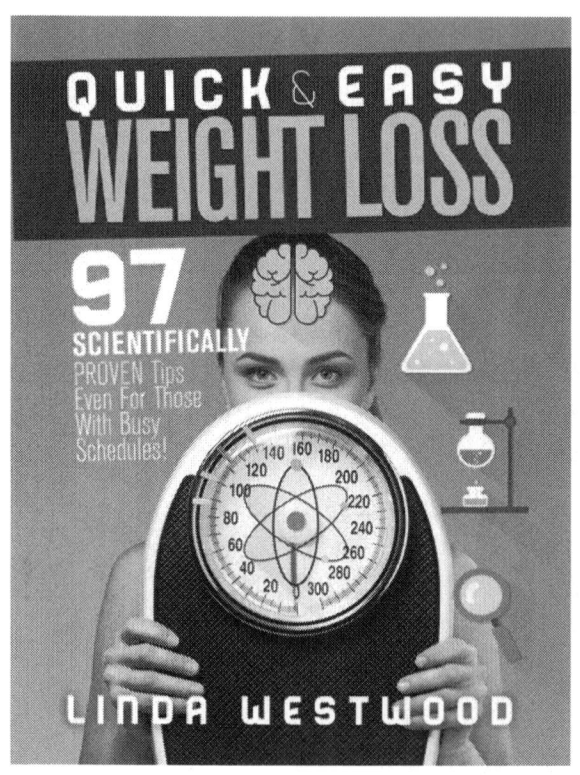

To download your FREE book, go to:

TopFitnessAdvice.com

Chapter 3: Health Benefits Associated with 5:2 Diet Plan

With a balanced fasting your digestive system will get a rest and it will work longer and in a better way.

With the help of 5:2 diet plan you can change your daily eating habits for good and remain fat free for lifelong. Once you have reduced you have a control on your weight you can fast for one day and maintain a constant weight. Fasting days might sound difficult but you will get used to this within a few weeks and then you will feel very light for the day without showing any signs of lethargy.

This diet plan reduces your risk of getting any kind of chronic diseases like diabetes type two and more. The diet plan also prohibits the growth of IGF-1 hormone in our body. It is this hormone which accelerates ageing of human body and for some also leads to cancer.

The diet plan is quite simple and flexible and you can continue with this plan for a longer duration because you can enjoy your favorite dishes without feeling guilty about them.

Chapter 4: Precautions and Extra Activities while Following 5:2 Diet Plan

If you are a diabetic patient then before undertaking 5:2 diet you should consult your doctor first. You can also consult a nutritionist and get your diet chart planned with the nutritionist's help. Pregnant women, children and people recovering from injuries should refrain from taking such diets.

If you feel fatigue and energy less in those two fasting days then again consult your doctor before carrying on with the diet plan.

5:2 diet plan is just the initial step towards getting a healthy body. If you want to get faster results, you will need to move a step ahead and do some kind of physical workout. You can start with gym, aerobics or any other form of exercise that suits you.

You should take proper sleep at night so that your metabolism and body clock works perfectly. This is necessary to get healthy results.

If you have any kind of bad habit like smoking and drinking then you should try and change these habits. You should also inculcate the habit of drinking a lot of water on a daily basis. This ensures that all your body waste is excreted out.

In a 5:2 diet plan, it is important to take care of the calorie count during those 5 days. It is easy to miss the target, especially when you have fasted the previous day. If you keep a check on your diet for the rest of non-fasting days, you will witness results within no time.

Chapter 5: 2 Days Fasting Recipes for Breakfast and Snacks

You should never skip your breakfast just because you are on a strict diet plan; rather it is important to maintain a balanced diet. You just need to plan your breakfast right.

Devise a diet plan where you can get energy for morning chores and also you intake only 100 calories. We are giving you a few delicious recipes that will suffice your purpose. You can also do a bit of mix and match according to your needs.

Greek Yogurt, Blueberry Kiwi Smoothie

It contains 95 calories in total. You might not love the taste of the recipe but it gives you a lot of anti-oxidants.

Ingredients

- 1 Kiwi, chopped

- 3 tbsp Greek yogurt, fat free

- 1.75 Oz blueberries

Method

1. You can take a bowl, mix all the three ingredients and have a sweet breakfast in morning.

2. You can take the three ingredients in a grinder bowl and grind it. Drink it in a form of smoothie.

Bread with Honey

If you need a break of sweet in between your diet plan then you can pour some honey on a slice of bread and enjoy a perfect combination of soft bread with light honey. The recipe contains a total of 95 calories.

Ingredients

- 1 slice of wheat bread

- 2 tbsp honey

Method

1. Take the bread slice and apply honey evenly on the slice. Fold the slice from centre and have the perfect morning sandwich.

Mushrooms with Eggs

You have to make scrambled eggs but without adding any butter or milk in it. Eggs contain a lot of proteins and you will feel full till afternoon time. Mushrooms add a crispy texture and bulk to the dish. It contains 91 calories.

Ingredients

- 1 medium size egg

- 100 grams Chopped mushroom

Method

1. Take a non-stick pan and pour egg contents in it.

2. Keep stirring the contents till it becomes dry.

3. Add mushroom at the end and have a sumptuous breakfast.

Spinach Omelette

This dish is a perfect way of getting proteins and iron in your morning time. Iron ensures that your hemoglobin level is maintained and protein helps in building your body muscle, which automatically reduces fat.

Ingredients

- 1 egg

- 50 grams chopped spinach

- Salt, pepper and herbs to taste

Method

1. Take a bowl and whisk egg contents in the bowl.

2. Pour the content on griller frying pan and spread the content evenly on pan.

3. Let the omelette cook nicely from bottom and then add chopped spinach from the top.

4. Cook omelette from both the side.

5. Sprinkle some salt, pepper and herbs on top of spinach to add extra flavor to your delicious breakfast.

Fruity Yogurt

Yogurt contains protein, probiotics, B12, iodine and calcium. All these elements keep you healthy and strong. Iodine, especially, keeps a check on fat around your belly area. It is a great slimming factor. When you combine several mineral rich fruits with it, then this becomes a wholesome dish for you. The dish contains 96 calories.

Ingredients

- 50 grams raspberries

- 50 grams strawberries

- 50 grams blackberries

- 1 apricot

- 3 tbsp Greek yogurt

Method

1. Make thin segments of apricot and chop all the berries that you have.

2. Take a bowl and mix all the ingredients nicely. Enjoy the delicious yogurt.

Honey Porridge

This is one dish that will give some carb boost to your morning. We are making porridge with oats that will keep your full. You can have this recipe when you have a hectic planned morning time. We have also substituted milk with water, which will keep a check on total calorie count.

The dish contains a total of 99 calories. If you are taking less of oats then you can add some nuts and add extra taste to the dish without increasing calorie count.

Ingredients

- ¼ tbsp honey

- 30 grams porridge oats

- ¼ tsp cinnamon

- Water as required

Method

1. Take a bowl and mix porridge oats and honey in the bowl.

2. Mix some water in the bowl to get a good consistency of the dish.

3. Sprinkle cinnamon from top and mix well.

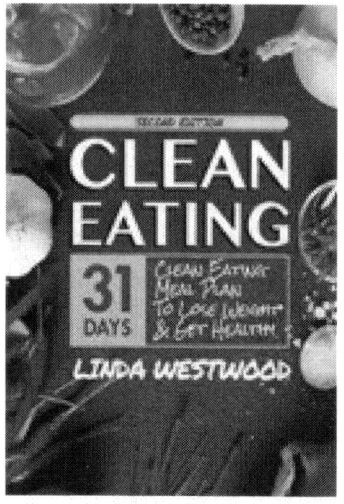
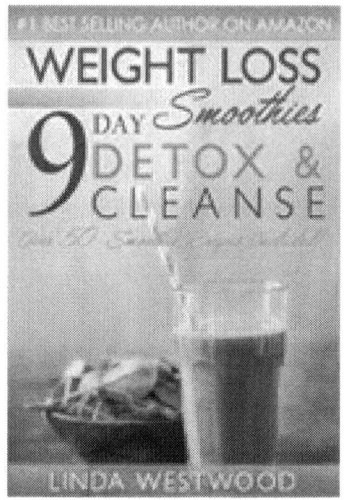
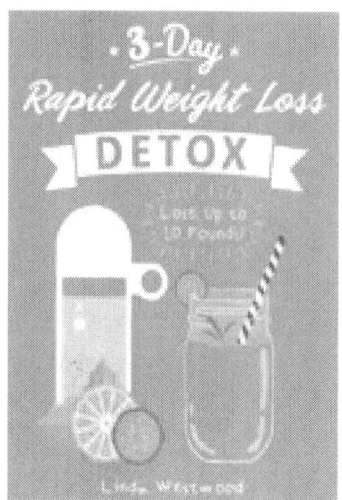
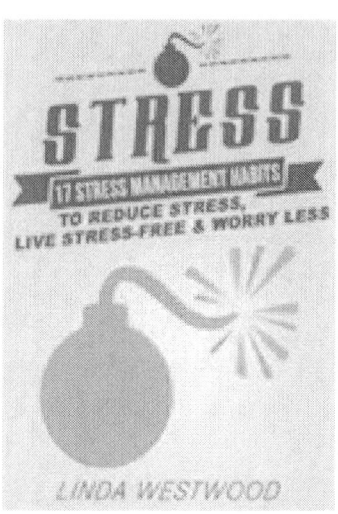

Check out Linda's best selling books at:

TopFitnessAdvice.com/go/books

Beans Toast

Beans will not increase the calorie count of your breakfast and will add a different taste to your usual routine breakfast. The dish is healthy and is very easy to make. The dish contains a total of 97 calories.

Ingredients

- 1 slice of whole wheat bread

- 50 grams of baked beans

Method

1. Take the bread slice and put it in toaster.

2. Take out bean from a can and heat it in microwave.

3. Apply bean on top of toast and have a delicious breakfast.

Ham Omelette

This dish will make you happy because we have a perfect combination of ham and egg in breakfast for you. This is a dish full of proteins and will keep a smile on your face for the whole day long. This dish contains a total of 97 calories.

Ingredients

- 1 egg

- 1 thin ham slice

- Salt and pepper to taste

Method

1. Take a bowl and whisk egg contents properly.

2. Take the ham slice and chop it finely.

3. Take a frying pan and pour whisked egg on the pan.

4. Spread chopped ham evenly on omelette.

5. Sprinkle salt and pepper according to your taste and have a fulfilling breakfast.

Chapter 6: 2 Days Fasting Recipes for Lunch and Dinner

Controlling your calorie intake during lunch time becomes a bit difficult. It is mid-day and you are basically exhausted with your morning chores. You feel like enjoying a delicious meal without worrying about calorie intake.

We have some good recipes for you that will ensure that your lunch is delicious, you fell full and your calorie intake is below 200 calories, as required under your 5:2 diet plan.

You can have soups, salads and even potatoes; just ensure you take right quantity in right form.

Leek Soup with Saffron Twist

This soup recipe is perfect for your lunch time. It is tasty, crunchy and full of proteins. You can pack it in your lunch box or even store it in freezer for future use. You can have this soup with a crunchy bread toast, but just keep your calories on check. This soup contains a total of 134 calories.

Ingredients

- 100 grams leek

- ¼ cup chopped onion

- 8 grams butter

- ¼ vegetable stock cubes

- 70 grams peeled and chopped potato

- 25 grams peas

- Oil for frying

- A pinch of saffron

- 1/4tbsp flour

- ¼ egg white

Method

1. Take a pan and heat oil in it.

2. Fry onions in the pan for about 10 minutes and add 90 grams sliced leek in the pan.

3. Pour ¼ liters of water in this pan and bring it to boil.

4. Add vegetable stock cube and potato in the pan, and cook the ingredients for about 10 minutes.

5. Add peas and cook all the ingredients for 10 minutes.

6. Take another bowl, whisk egg white, flour and saffron in the bowl. Make a thick batter from this.

7. Cut 10 grams left out leeks into rings and dip them into the flour batter.

8. Cook leek rings on a dry frying pan.

9. Take soup in a bowl and garnish it with leek rings.

Colorful Cabbage Salad

This salad recipe is perfect for a light lunch. The recipe also contains pumpkin seeds which adds a protein punch to the recipe. Other seasoning like fennel and mustard adds a different flavor to the whole recipe. The dish contains 129 calories in total.

Ingredients

- 1/2tbs sunflower oil

- ¼ red onion sliced

- 50 grams shredded red cabbage

- 30 grams pointed cabbage

- ¼ small grated carrot

- 1tsp toasted pumpkin seeds

- ¼ cup parsley

- 1/4tsp wholegrain mustard

- A pinch of brown sugar

- 1/4tsp balsamic vinegar

- 1 tsp olive oil

Method

1. Take a frying pan and heat some oil in the pan.

2. Add onion and fennel in the pan and cook both the ingredients for 2 minutes.

3. Add red cabbage and cook everything for another 3 minutes.

4. Take the contents in a bowl and add raw carrot and cabbage in the bowl.

5. Take another bowl and whisk mustard, pumpkin seeds, olive oil, sugar, vinegar and parsley nicely.

6. Serve the seasoning on the cabbage salad and have a nice lunch.

Steak and Orange Salad

You can make this tender and tangy salad within 30 minutes. This is a perfect recipe for a sunny afternoon, with a hectic evening schedule. You can have this salad individually or can side it with a whole wheat bread slice. This dish contains 179 calories.

Ingredients

- 1.5 tbsp olive oil

- 40 grams sirloin steak, pieces

- ¼ orange segment

- ¼ orange juice

- ½ tbsp sherry vinegar

- ½ tsp mustard

- 2 wedges of onion

- ½ chicory cut into 2 pieces length wise

Method

1. Take steak pieces and rub oil on both the sides of each piece.

2. Take a fry pan and cook all steak pieces on both the sides for about 2 minute.

3. Wrap all the pieces in a foil and set it aside.

4. Take another pan and boil orange juice in it till it is reduced till half.

5. Add vinegar, mustard and ½ tsp of oil in the orange juice.

6. Add red onion in the oil and cook it till becomes brown in color.

7. Mix all the ingredients in the orange sauce and serve it on plate with red chicory as garnishing.

Chicken Pita

Chicken pitta is a delicious dish that is perfect for a weekend family get together. Even kids love this delicious recipe for their lunch box. Also, you will consume only 162 calories in one chicken pitta serving.

Ingredients

- ½ tbsp natural yogurt

- ½ tsp tomato puree

- ½ tsp curry paste

- 40 grams chicken strips

- 1/4tsp vegetable oil

- 1 pita bread

- 1 tbsp shredded lettuce

- 1 Cherry tomato

Method

1. Take a bowl and mix yogurt, curry paste and tomato puree in it.

2. Toss chicken pieces in the bowl and cover all sides of chicken with paste.

3. Cover chicken and put it in freeze for about 15 minutes.

4. Take a non-stick pan and heat oil in the pan.

5. Cook marinated chicken pieces in the pan for about 8 minutes but ensure chicken piece is still juicy.

6. Take pitta bread and open it.

7. Fill pitta bread with shredded lettuce and chicken pieces in it.
8. Top pitta bread with cherry tomatoes and serve it hot.

A Special Gift Just For YOU

FOR A LIMITED TIME ONLY – Get Linda's best-selling book *"Quick & Easy Weight Loss: 97 Scientifically Proven Tips Even For Those With Busy Schedules!"* absolutely FREE!

Readers who have read this bonus book along with this book have seen the greatest changes in their weight loss both *FAST & EASILY* and have improved overall fitness levels – so it is *highly recommended* to get this bonus book.

Once again, as a big thank-you for downloading this book, I'd like to offer it to you *100% FREE for a LIMITED TIME ONLY!*

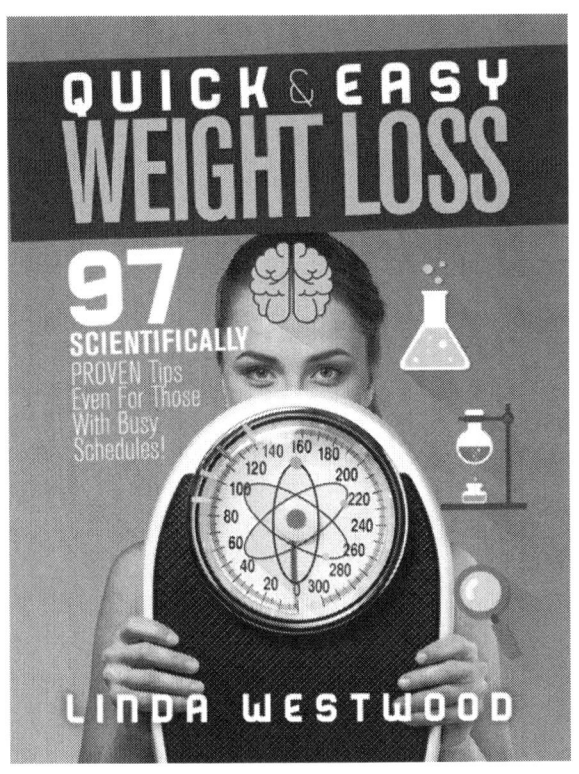

To download your FREE book, go to:

TopFitnessAdvice.com

Chapter 7: 5 Days Fasting Recipes

In the earlier recipes you get to know what all you can have in 2 days of fasting. In this section we will give you recipes that you can have in rest 5 days where you are supposed to have about below 2000 calories per day (2500 for men).

We will give you recipes that are healthy and tasty. You will be amazed to know that we have recipes like pasta and meatballs in store for you. It is not necessary to always have soups and salads when you are on a diet.

Fish Filo Pastry

Make your fish dish a special one with a crunchy twist in it with the help of filo pastry. With fish you can get a lot of iodine and remain healthy. The dish contains 463 calories.

Ingredients

- 2 filo pastry sheet

- 2tbsp chopped onion

- 1/2 small bay leaf

- 80ml fish stock

- 12ml white wine

- 120 grams mixed fish like salmon, scallop and raw prawn

- 8 grams plain flour

- 12grams butter

- 25ml fresh cream

- 1tsp lemon zest

- 1 tbsp chopped parsley

- 1 small deseeded and quartered tomato

- Salt and pepper as per taste

Method

1. Take a pan, add stock, wine, bay leaf and onion in it and boil all contents for about 5 minutes.

2. Add large pieces of fish first and add other small pieces after 2 minutes and cook all the content for about 3 more minutes.

3. Take pieces of fish out from the pan and out it in a baking tray.
4. Reheat all the drippings and reduce it will 600 ml and remove bay leaf from it.

5. Take a bowl and mix half of butter and flour in the bowl and make a paste out of it.

6. Add small spoons of mixture in the dripping pan and make a sauce after heating it for 2 minutes.

7. Add cream, lemon zest, parsley, tomato puree, tomato and seasoning in the pan, and at last add fish.

8. Take a filo pastry and brush butter on top of it.

9. Add the sauce and add another sheet on the top with edges tugged in.

10. Bake this dish for 25 minutes at 200 degrees C and serve it hot.

Chili Meatballs

It is always good to have some chili food when you are on a diet plan. At first, they increase the heat within your body which increases the burning down of fat. Secondly, it brings a good change to your usual dull food routine. This dish contains a total of 371 calories.

Ingredients

- 125 grams beef chunks

- 8 grams chili con spice mix

- 1/2 grated small onion

- Cooking spray

- ¼ small chili sliced

- 1 tsp tomato puree

- 200 grams chopped tomato

- 40 ml beef stock

- 100 grams black been

- Salt and pepper as per taste

Method

1. Take a bowl and mix beef, chili mix and onion in it and make 6 balls from the mixture.

2. Take a pan and spray some cooking oil in it and fry all the 6 balls from all the sides for about 10 minutes.

3. Take another pan and heat some cooking oil in it.

4. Add chili, rest of the spice mix and tomato puree and cook for about 1 minute.

5. Add stock and tomatoes to the pan and cook over low flame for 10 minutes.

6. Add meatballs and beans in this pan and cook for another 5 minutes till the sauce becomes thicker.

7. You can serve hot meat balls with some brown rice and enjoy your fiesta.

Chicken Pasta

It is an easy dish and you can treat your family with a low calorie yet delicious dish. The dish contains a total of 426 calories.

Ingredients

- 85 grams pasta

- 45 grams peas

- 45 grams cooked chicken chunks

- 1/2tsp cream

- 1 tbsp chopped parsley

- Salt and pepper as per taste

Method

1. Cook pasta as per instructed in the packet.

2. Just before the pasta is fully cooked, 3 minutes before, add peas to the boiling pan.

3. Drain the two ingredients and shift it to a pan.

4. Add chicken, parsley and cream in the pan.

5. Put the pan over medium flame and cook everything for 2 minutes.

6. Sprinkle salt and pepper from the top.

Cod Nuggets and Wedged Sweet Potato

Fish fingers are good for your taste buds as well as for your health. To make this recipe healthier, we have added a flavor of sweet potato chips instead of normal ones. This dish has a total of 480 calories.

Ingredients

- 1 cod filled chunked

- 1/2tbsp plain flour

- ½ egg beaten

- 25 grams wheat bread crumbs

- 8ml olive oil

- ½ sweet potato cut into wedges

- 4ml honey

- Sunflower oil

- Sour cream

Method

1. Take a piece of cod, cover it in flour, dip it in beaten egg and then make a final coat of bread crumbs.

2. Cover all the pieces and put it in freeze for about 20 minutes.

3. Take a roasting tin and heat olive oil for about 4 minutes and add sweet potatoes in it.

4. Roast the cod in tin for about 20 minutes by turning it up and down.

5. Brush the pieces with honey and cook it till it becomes tender in oven for about 10 minutes.

6. Take a fry pan and heat sunflower oil in it.

7. Fry fish pieces on all the sides in the pan for about 3 minutes.

8. Drain oil with the help of tissue paper and serve it with sweet potato wedges.

Thai Noodles

There is something special about all the Thai dishes. The special Thai ingredients give a very different taste to normal noodles. All the ingredients are readily available because of which you can make this dish is a very less time. This dish contains a total of 307 calories.

Ingredients

- ¾ tbsp Thai curry paste

- 90 gram Butternut squash and sweet potato

- 55ml coconut milk

- ½ vegetable stock cubes

- 34 grams frozen peas

- 50 grams readymade noodles

- 1/3rd pak choi head

- Basil leaves

- Red chili

Method

1. Take a large pan and add Thai paste and butternut sweet potato squash in the pan.

2. Stir fry all the contents for about 2 minutes on medium heat.

3. Add coconut milk and hot water in the pan.

4. Add stock cubes in the pan and simmer all the contents for about 15 minutes till all the vegetables get tender.

5. Add peas to the pan, add noodles and let all the ingredients simmer for about 2 minutes.

6. Take pak choi and pour hot water in it.
7. Serve curry in bowls along with pak choi.

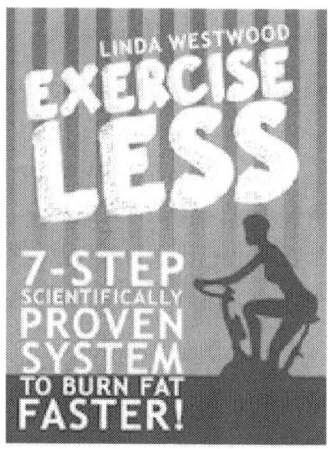
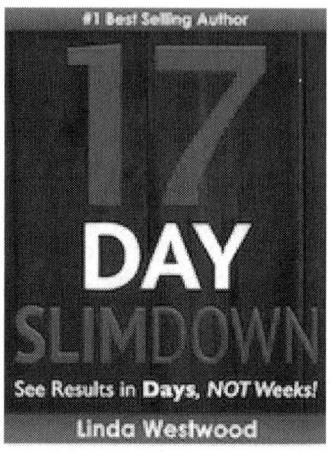
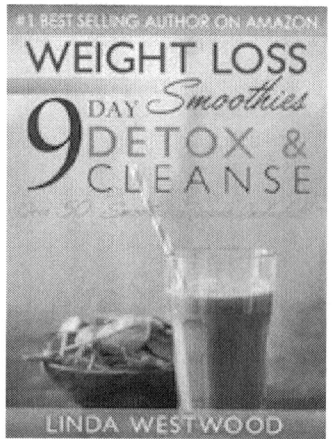
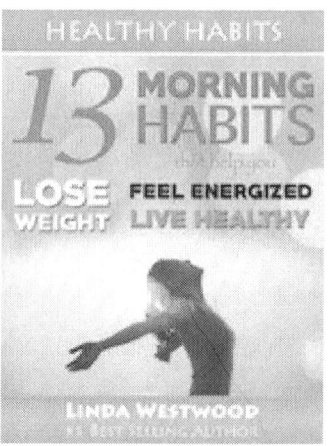

Check out Linda's best selling books at:

TopFitnessAdvice.com/go/books

Chapter 8: Powerful Diet Plans That Work

Your body needs calories on a daily basis, which you get from the food you take on a daily basis. When the amount of calorie that your body needs exceeds the amount you intake then your body starts using the stored energy. This stored energy is fats. If your body suffers from this deficiency for a long time, then you start reducing your body weight and fat. This is however, a basic explanation.

There are two sources of energy for body, on a daily basis; carbohydrates and fats. For some, metabolism works perfectly well when we limit their calorie intake. For some, the count of calorie does not matter because their body energy depends heavily on the carbohydrate levels. When their carbohydrate intake is decreased, they automatically reduce weight. Atkins weight plan follow the second technique.

There is another diet plan, 7 days diet plan, which produces great affect on human body. In this you are supposed to eat a specific diet for each day for a total of seven days, where you get to eat a mixture of fruits, salads, milk and rice.

In this plan, basically you reduce the intake of carbohydrate and give a continuous supply of protein to your body. This protein goes into building muscle in your body, which in turn decreases the stored fat content of your body. Also, you cleanse you body over 7 days with a continuous supply of fibers and minerals, which again helps in decreasing fat content of body.

You should know what kind of plan will suit your body and you should accordingly follow a plan. To make your 5:2 diet work well we are giving you some truly exciting recipes with the help of which you will not even feel that you are on a diet plan, and yet it will show results on your body.

Final Words

I would like to thank you for downloading my book and I hope I have been able to help you and educate you about something new.

If you have enjoyed this book and would like to share your positive thoughts, could you please take 30 seconds of your time to go back and give me a review on my Amazon book page!

I greatly appreciate seeing these reviews because it helps me share my hard work!

Again, thank you and I wish you all the best with your cooking journey!

Last Chance to Get YOUR Bonus!

FOR A LIMITED TIME ONLY – Get Linda's best-selling book *"Quick & Easy Weight Loss: 97 Scientifically Proven Tips Even For Those With Busy Schedules!"* absolutely FREE!

Readers who have read this bonus book along with this book have seen the greatest changes in their weight loss both *FAST & EASILY* and have improved overall fitness levels – so it is *highly recommended* to get this bonus book.

Once again, as a big thank-you for downloading this book, I'd like to offer it to you *100% FREE for a LIMITED TIME ONLY!*

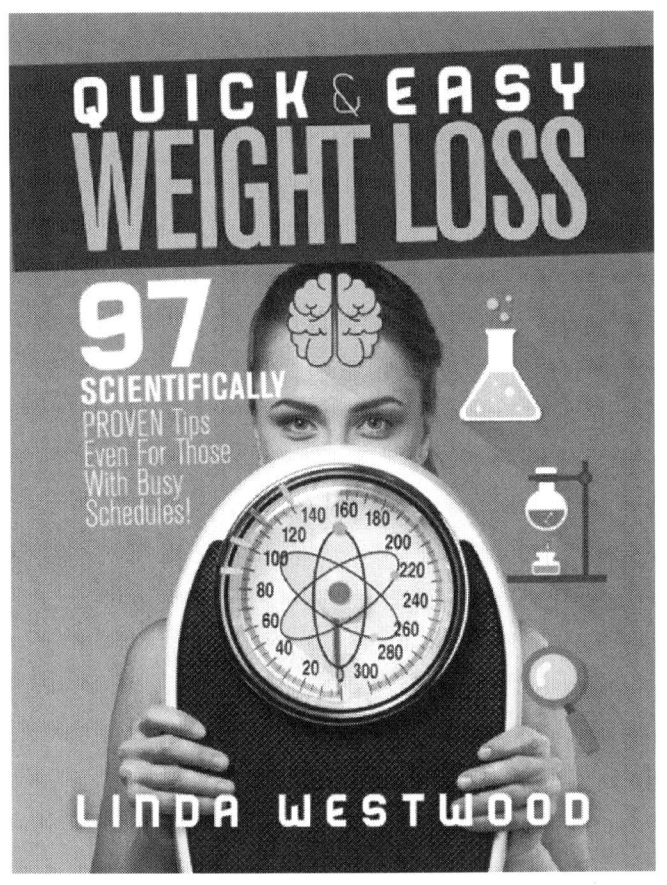

To download your FREE book, go to:

TopFitnessAdvice.com

Sneak Peek
13 Morning Habits to Lose Weight

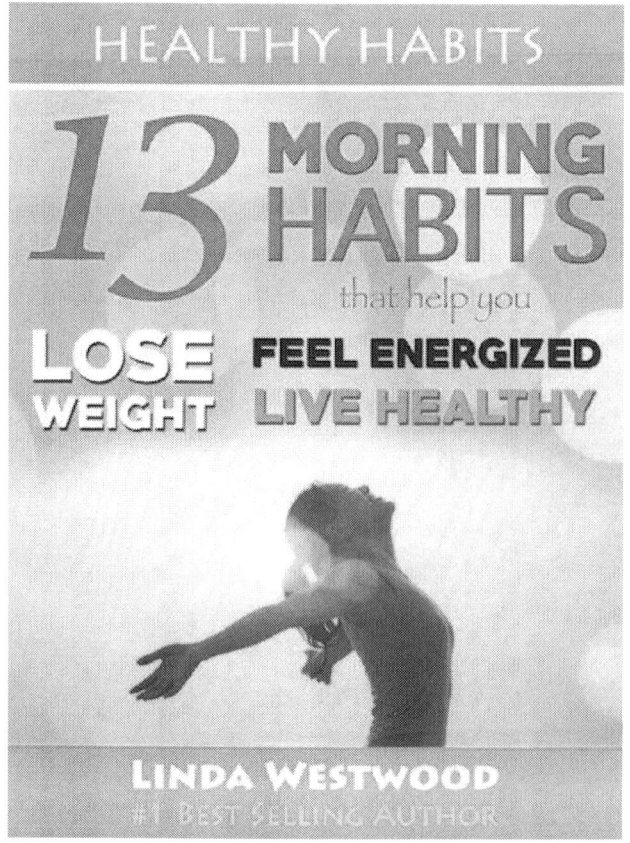

Buy this book TODAY at:

TopFitnessAdvice.com/go/books

Who is this book for?

Have you tried to lose weight before but failed?

Are you struggling to stick to healthy habits?

Are you one of those people who *know* what to do, but struggle to *actually do* it?

Then this book is for you!

I am going to share with you some of the MOST effective morning habits that you can add into your life to lose weight, feel great and be energized throughout your entire day!

I have given you a simple action plan at the end of each chapter so you can implement each habit very easily!

Also, you don't have to be overweight to benefit from these habits.

Yes, they help you lose weight, but they also help you live a healthy life, as well as feel recharged and energized ALL DAY LONG!

What will this book teach you?

This book is not like others!

It doesn't just contain generic advice that we all already know, but actual morning habits that have been identified to INCREASE weight loss, IMPROVE energy levels, and LEAD to a more healthy life!

Some of these habits are very simple and you can begin implementing them from tomorrow morning, and some are a little more difficult, in that you will need to practice them more!

I will also share with you why each of these habits work and are so effective – along with a simple action plan to help get you started and on your way to lasting success!

Introduction

Want to lose weight and feel great?

Then this is the book for you.

If you are anything like me, you have tried just about every diet on the planet and have lost and regained weight several times over.

It's a vicious cycle – you diet and lose the fat, only to find that it arrives back with MORE when the diet is over!

Diets don't work!

They create an unnatural feeling of deprivation and the body starts to rebel quite fast.

I, for example, am not a choc-a-holic – I enjoy chocolates, but don't eat too many of them… until I go on a diet.

Once I start a diet my body starts demanding chocolates, and all the other stuff I shouldn't be eating.

Many people find that the same type of thing happens to them. Dieting is clearly not the answer. If dieting did work, there would only be one diet plan out there and no one would be overweight or obese.

This book is different – it is not a diet book.

In this book I give you 13 little habits that you can add into your lifestyle so that you naturally and painlessly lose weight and keep it off.

Thirteen may seem like a lot but here's the rub – you will adopt each one individually, at your own pace. In fact, I insist that you do not rush it – this process should take no less than two weeks at the very least.

I know that you are motivated to get started on everything now, but this program works because it is done step-by-step. Introducing each habit individually allows your body to cope more readily with the changes. Try to do them all at once and you will probably give up.

Each habit will, by itself, help you to lose weight. As you build more habits in, each habit builds on the last and you will see even more progress.

Some habits will be easier to adopt than others but, at the end of the day, it is worthwhile to adopt all of them.

Eventually, when you have adopted all the habits, you will be living at the next level – you'll be healthier and more energetic in ways that you have never been before.

Read the book slowly, I have written out an action plan for each habit to make it easy for you.

No more excuses – let's dive right in!

Morning Habit #1 – The MOST Common Habit Of Healthy People

The most common habit of healthy people is that they wake up early every morning.

Your body will thank you for it – our bodies were designed to sleep when it is nighttime and to be awake during the day when the sun is up. Getting up earlier, around the time the sun rises, is more in sync with our natural circadian rhythms.

You will find that you settle into this sleep cycle a lot easier as time goes by, resulting in the right amounts of rest each night.

The Leptin and Ghrelin Issue

Remember the last time you got to bed too late and woke up feeling less than refreshed.

Perhaps it was last night?

How hungry did you feel?

How easy was it to make healthy eating choices or did you just want to eat everything in sight?

Better sleep leaves you more able to deal with the stresses of the day. By not getting enough sleep, you are putting stress on your body and more cortisol is produced.

More cortisol means two of the hormones that help regulate appetite – Leptin and Ghrelin – begin to function ineffectively.

Not only are you more vulnerable to poor eating choices because you are tired, but your brain is not getting the right hunger messages from the hormones that it should.

Your brain is demanding energy and wants high calorie foods to satisfy it. Ghrelin is suppressed so the brain is not sent the message that you have eaten enough.

When you get enough sleep, your brain does not have this need for instant energy since your cortisol levels are a lot more stable. You will therefore find it a lot easier to follow a healthier eating plan and make good choices.

Even your metabolic rate benefits – those who get enough sleep have a much stronger metabolism.

According to this article in Women's Health magazine, studies have proven conclusively that being exposed to morning light by waking up earlier is linked to a decreased chance of being overweight.

Try it yourself – go to be tonight with your curtains open and let the sun wake you in the morning.

I'm a Night Owl

This may seem a little tough at first, especially for the night owls, but it won't take long before you get used to it.

It was even hard for me at first!

But what you do need to realize is that you are doing this so that you can live life to the fullest.

I figured that it came down to a simple choice – either I was happy being overweight and could carry on hitting the snooze button or I was willing to feel miserable for a few days so that I could feel great for the rest of my life.

Basically you need to figure out whether or not the payoff for staying up late and waking up late is really worth not giving this its best chance.

ACTION PLAN

1. This is best started immediately. If you have a big day coming up or are worried about being tired, schedule it to start over a weekend instead.

2. Decide on what time is early in your part of the world and count back 8 hours from there. This is your new target bedtime.

3. About an hour before bedtime, you want to switch off your laptop, TV and cell phone. If possible, dim the lights in the house. (If you don't have a dimmer, wear a pair of sunglasses – yes, seriously!) Artificial light is very stimulating to the brain and interferes with your body's production of melatonin – the hormone that makes you sleepy.

4. Do something relaxing leading up to bedtime like reading a book – just not a best seller.

5. Go to bed when you are feeling sleepy – if you do not fall asleep within about 15 minutes either get up and start reading again (don't forget the sunglasses) or, if you are able to, just relax in bed. It is important not to get caught up in how much sleep you are getting.

6. Set the alarm early and disable the snooze button.

7. When the alarm goes off, jump out of bed, open your curtains and bask in the sunlight. If possible, go outside for five minutes as well.

Morning Habit #2 – The Morning Drink That Will Change Your Life

The next one is super easy.

Drink warm lemon water first thing in the morning – use water that is tepid, not boiling, and use fresh lemons.

The Benefits:

- **<u>Smoother Digestion</u>**

  Because of its chemical make-up, it stimulates the liver into producing bile – the acid that we need for digestion. This benefits the digestive tract even further by helping to get rid of internal toxins. Contrary to popular belief, lemon is not acidic in the digestive tract and can help treat heartburn, bloating and belching. For those with dread diseases, lemon water can help to gently get their bowel movements back on track.

- **<u>Detoxifier/Diuretic</u>**

  Part of the reason that it is a valuable detoxifier is that it is a diuretic – you may urinate more allowing your body to get rid of toxins faster. This also benefits your urinary tract. It doesn't stop there – it also helps to detoxify the liver.

- **<u>Weight Loss</u>**

The pectin in lemons is a fiber and this is great for killing hunger pangs. Those who eat a diet that is richer in fiber, and thus richer in alkaline, actually find it easier to lose weight.

- **Boost Your Immune System**

The high Vitamin C content makes them valuable in treating and preventing colds and flu. The high potassium content helps with the brain and nerves and also with regulating blood pressure. The Vitamin C also has anti-inflammatory effects. Overall, they are great weapons in the fight against disease.

- **Alkaline Properties**

As mentioned before, lemon juice becomes alkaline in the blood stream. Drink it often and the blood's pH becomes less acidic. This, in turn, helps to protect you against diseases, as they require an acidic pH to thrive. If you have gout, lemon juice can help neutralize it.

- **Glowing Skin**

The nutritional content of the juice helps to nourish the skin and also helps to fight of free radicals. It could also help fight the bacteria that cause acne. With less toxins circulating in your system, you can expect clearer skin as well.

- It is a well-known fact that the citrus oils in aromatherapy are stimulating. Whilst the smell of the juice in the water is not as intense, it can still give you a bit of a mood-enhancing boost.

- The juice also helps to kill off the bacteria in the mouth that cause problems. That said, the acidity in the lemon can affect the tooth enamel so you should rinse out your mouth after drinking it and wait a while before brushing your teeth.

- The water helps to up your hydration levels thereby increasing your energy levels. It is a great way to brush the cobwebs of sleep from your brain.

This is such an easy fix that it is amazing that it does actually work. Grow your own lemon tree if you can – that way you have fresh fruit on demand all the time.

ACTION PLAN

1. You will need half a fresh lemon a day, so unless you have a lemon tree in your garden, get a few. (No more than 4 – they are better fresh).

2. As soon as you have said hello to the sun, pour yourself a glass of tepid water – not too hot or too cold, just right!

3. Cut your lemon in half and reserve one half for tomorrow. Squeeze as much juice as you can manage from the other one.

4. Bottoms up! I find that downing it is best. I have a sweet tooth so I didn't enjoy it at first – you quickly get used to it. Now I can feel the difference if I skip my lemon water.

Did You Enjoy 13 Morning Habits?

Buy this book TODAY at:

TopFitnessAdvice.com/go/books

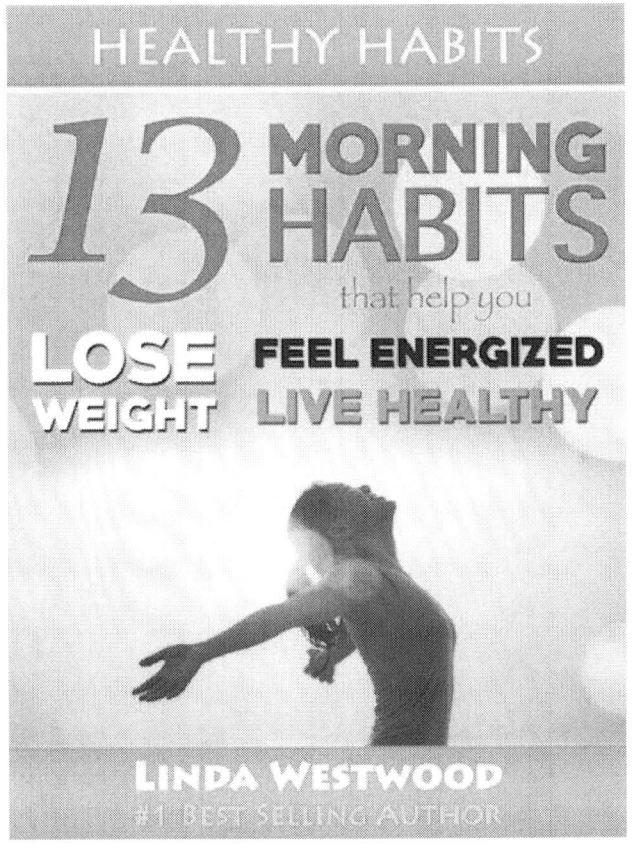

Sneak Peek
3 Day Rapid Weight Loss Detox

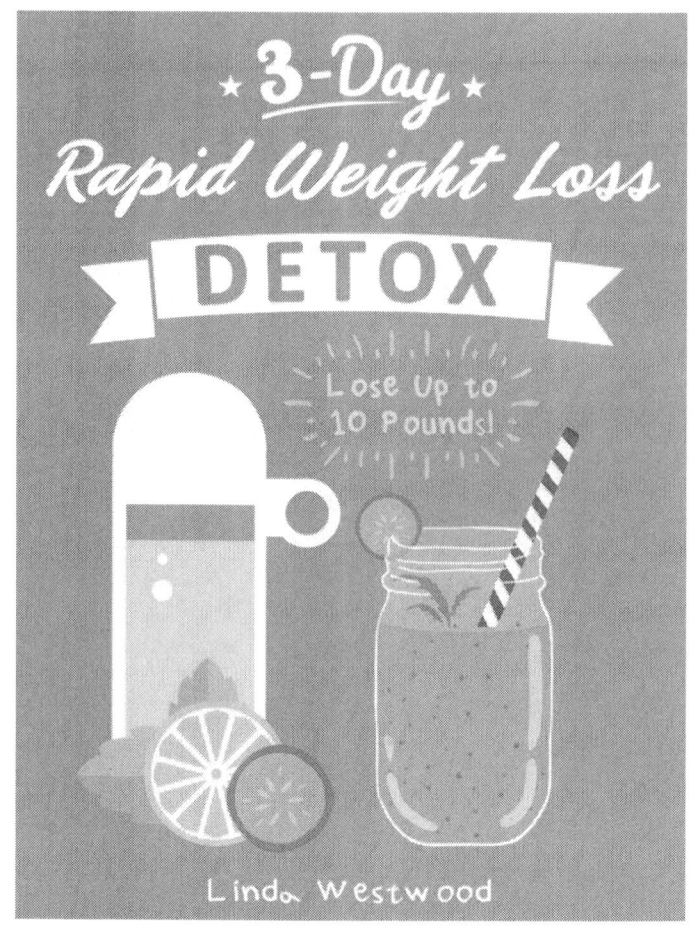

Buy this book TODAY at:

TopFitnessAdvice.com/go/books

Who is this book for?

Do you need a *strong* kick-start with your weight loss?

Do you need to lost weight *FAST*?

Do you have an event coming up that you need to *shed pounds fast* for?

If you answered "Yes" to any of those questions – **this book is for you!**

I am going to share with you the most effective way to rapidly lose weight and detox your mind and body in just 3 days!

I have put it all together in this awesome Weekend Weight Loss plan!

The best part about is that you are going to see amazing results and this will *TRANSFORM YOUR BODY (inside and outside) IN JUST 3 DAYS*!

You can be a complete beginner or someone who works out regularly, it doesn't matter!

If this sounds like it could help you, then keep reading…

What will this book teach you?

Inside, I will teach you one of the best ways to quickly lose weight, especially targeted to cleansing your body with a 3-day detox!

You will feel the healthiest you have ever felt – have the most energy you have ever had – and the fat will be melting *constantly!*

How?

Because you're going to be consuming the right things to cleanse your body in a short period of time.

In this book, I give you the plan right in front of you that will change your life – all you have to do is follow it!

One of the most important things for you to realize when reading this book is that this weight loss plan *really does work!*

However…

For you to achieve *real success*, you HAVE to apply this to your life.

This is where most people fail – they read through the entire book but do nothing.

You MUST try your best to apply as you read through the book!

Introduction

Are you struggling to lose weight?

You are not alone. 30 percent of the world's population is overweight or obese.

Why does it matter?

What makes millions of people endeavor to lose weight each year?

Frankly, health. Obesity can lead to high blood pressure, diabetes, osteoarthritis, heart disease and coronary artery disease, fatty liver, sleep apnea, and certain kinds of cancer.

Many people who begin a weight loss regimen do not continue because even when they eat a healthy diet and exercise they cannot seem to lose weight.

However, if you are losing the battle of the bulge, the problem might not be your diet. It might be within your body itself.

Slow Metabolism

Metabolism refers to the efficiency with which your body burns calories for energy. The "speed" of your metabolism, whether it is fast or slow, coincides with the ease of losing weight.

Many factors can have an effect of the speed of your metabolism. Your fitness level and your body composition, that is the ratio of muscle to fat, will affect it. If you carry more muscle, you burn calories more quickly.

Your age has tremendous influence on your metabolism. When you are young, you have a speedy metabolism that burns off calories very quickly.

Do you look back longingly at your teenage years when you could eat anything and not gain weight?

You were able to eat like that because your metabolism was lightning fast. But, as you age your metabolism slows down.

Even in your 20s your metabolism can stay pretty fast and keep you slim. But after you turn 30 your metabolism slows down a lot and that can lead to weight gain.

Your metabolism will continue to slow down as you age. So, unless you find a solution that works for you, it will just get more and more difficult to lose weight.

It is, however, possible to speed it back up, and your detox is a good precursor to the healthy lifestyle that will do just that.

Body Pollution

Another factor that can make it hard to lose weight is years of body pollution.

All that fast food, refined sugar, and extra calories can take a huge toll on your body. Your liver, which is what processes wastes in the body, may not continue functioning effectively because it's been working overtime.

When you eat an unhealthy diet, fail to exercise and do not take care of yourself for years at a time, your body suffers. The effects of all those harmful years can make your body sluggish and polluted, which can make it tough to lose weight.

Detox and Weight Loss

If you want to kick start weight loss or cleanse your body so that it functions as effectively as possible, a detox is the way to go.

Detox is short for detoxification, and it is the process by which we remove toxins from our systems. Participating in a detox can be less than pleasant, but it will rejuvenate your body, clean out the pollution and toxins, and make it easier for you to lose weight.

Additionally, a liquid diet is effective for weight loss.

While the 3-day detox diet is designed only for use over a short time period, similar diets are used to lose tremendous amounts of weight, with a doctor's supervision.

There are many other weight loss programs that suggest two shakes a day and a "sensible" dinner. So it should come as no surprise that the 3-day detox diet, being completely liquid, can perform amazingly to assist you in losing up to 10 pounds in one short weekend.

Chapter One: Why It Works

What happens to cars that never have an oil change?

The build up of sludge will destroy the motor. The same thing happens in your body when you do not take care of yourself.

If you stopped showering tomorrow what would happen to your skin?

Dirt would build up. Pollutants from the environment would build up. Your skin would look terrible, with probable breakouts, even rashes.

Your skin would also *feel* terrible. It would be itchy. Bacteria and toxins would build up and might cause sores and infections. So to prevent that you shower and wash with soap frequently.

Detox does the same thing for your internal systems that showering does for your skin. Over the years, all those pollutants and bacteria and other toxic chemicals in your body build up. They slow down your body's waste disposal system and make it difficult for your body to function.

You may gain weight, or have a harder time losing weight. Additionally, you may frequently feel exhausted, or lethargic. It may seem as if you are moving in a fog all the time. If your liver isn't filtering toxins out of your body the way it should you might find yourself getting sick more often.

An Internal Cleansing

When you go on a detox, you are giving your body a break from the daily barrage of fat, sugar, and other unhealthy pollutants to which you subject it. At the same time that you are giving your body a rest from breaking down and processing unhealthy foods, you are feeding it with healthy foods, such as fruits, vegetables and nuts.

Those healthy foods, when combined as the 3-day detox diet explains, will flush the toxins and bacteria out of your organs, your bloodstream, and everywhere else in your body. This will get your circulation and waste disposal systems working at full capacity again.

Once your body is running on all cylinders again it will be able to break down fat for energy and you will start to lose weight. It will also get rid of all the excess waste and nasty debris in your body that could be keeping you from losing weight and feeling your best.

Think of your body as being a living machine. All machines need maintenance. You don't expect your car to run forever with no maintenance, so why do you expect it of yourself?

If you want your body to be a fat burning machine, sometimes you need to give it a little tune up so that it will work the way it is supposed to work. A detox is exactly the kind of maintenance that your body needs to begin metabolizing food more efficiently.

There are several additional benefits to your 3-day detox.

The 3-day detox diet may bolster your immune system. Once your waste disposal system is cleaned out, your focus on vitamin rich super foods should serve to supercharge your immune system.

The detox will improve the appearance and clarity of your skin. The epidermis, or skin, is the body's largest organ. Of course, the removal of toxins will reflect in your skin. Although you may experience patchy, itchy skin, or even an increase in breakouts at the beginning of the program, by the end of it you should see beautiful results.

The 3-day detox can help you regain your focus of mind. Some followers of the program say that detoxing cleared up fuzzy thinking and got their bodies and minds in balance.

Detoxing can give you healthier hair. Many people have said that removing the toxins from their bodies allowed their hair to grow faster and become healthier.

The 3-day detox can have anti-aging benefits. The build up of toxins is one of the major causes of the effects we think of as aging. The process of clearing out impurities tackles free radicals that cause us to look and feel older.

As you can see, the 3-day detox can deliver much more in addition to weight loss!

Chapter Two: Prepare Before The Weekend

The best way to do a 3-day detox is to pick a weekend that you can focus on yourself. You should plan on staying home for most of that weekend.

If you are doing the detox to lose weight before going to a wedding, a banquet, or another special occasion, it is a smart idea to do the detox a week in advance of the event. That will give you time to recover and look great at the event. Don't worry; you won't gain back the weight in a week.

Why Do It On A Weekend?

Doing the 3-day detox on a weekend is highly recommended. You probably should not attempt to drag yourself to work when you don't feel or look your best.

A detox is great for your body once it is done. However, you might feel cranky or even more sluggish and tired while you are actually engaged in the detox. This reaction is due to your body working overtime getting rid of so many toxins and other unhealthy pollutants from your system.

So plan on taking a 3-day weekend to do the detox. You deserve it!

Make it at a spa weekend for yourself. Get some movies that you have been wanting to watch, load up on books and magazines, and plan on staying in your pajamas and pampering yourself all weekend.

By the time the detox is done you will be rested, and you will feel great. You will also be up to ten pounds lighter and your skin will be glowing. You will look fabulous for that special event.

Shop In Advance

Once you have picked a weekend to focus on your 3-day detox, you should take the time to create a shopping list. You will want to get all the items that you will need to do the detox in advance.

Going to the store during the detox will just tempt you to buy and eat a bunch of unhealthy food, and you will likely not feel up to it. One of the most important elements of any healthy lifestyle change is planning ahead. Another is avoiding temptation!

So it is smarter to buy everything you are going to need ahead of time. That way you have no reason to go to the store and no excuse to go off of the detox diet. Making a complete shopping list ahead of time will also ensure that you have everything you need to do the detox.

Your health and the success of the 3-day detox depends upon following the plan, and you can only do that if you have all the ingredients.

Ordering Supplies

Shopping in advance will also make it easier to find the items that you need to do the detox properly. Of course, you will have no trouble finding things like fruit and vegetables at the grocery store.

However, you might have a hard time finding the supplements that you need, some of the additional ingredients for the detox drinks, and the essential oils that you need for a detox bath. Thinking and planning ahead ensures that you will know if you can buy what you need or if you'll have to order it.

If you discover that you live in an area where items like those listed above can be difficult to procure, you will probably have to order some of them online.

Start researching the best shopping sites for those items as soon as you pick the weekend that you want to do to the detox. Order immediately, so that they will arrive in time. Another benefit to this approach is that if you decide to do the detox again for another event you will already have those items on hand.

Buy Organic and Local

When you buy the fruits and vegetables that you will be eating on the detox make a special effort to buy organic or local vegetables and fruit.

You are doing this detox to make your body healthy, so do not start out by eating unhealthy GMO fruit and vegetables which may introduce more pollutants and toxins into your system.

Remember that you are what you eat. If you want to be healthy, you must eat healthy food. Treating yourself and spending a little bit of extra money for organic or local produce is worth it for this purpose.

Once your body has detoxed you should use the lessons you will learn and make an effort to eat higher quality foods. You know you should stay away from processed food, refined sugar, and high fructose corn syrup and the 3-day detox will get you started down that healthy path.

Organic food, especially locally grown organic food, is richer in nutrients than conventionally grown food. Organic food is not exposed to chemical pesticides and fertilizers, and so will not reintroduce the toxins you are trying to flush out with the 3-day detox.

Local foods in particular retain more vitamins and minerals simply because they fresher.

Where to Shop for Local and Organic Foods

If you have a local natural foods store or food co-op you should be able to find plenty of organic choices of fruit and vegetables there.

You may be able to find the supplements and other supplies that you need there as well. Many natural food stores and co-ops carry spices, supplements, teas, and even the essential oils that you will need for your relaxing detox baths.

Some communities have a program called Community Supported Agriculture, or farm sharing. If you belong to a farm share, you pay for a crate of locally grown organic vegetables and fruit and you pay the farmer directly.

Some require an up front payment for a season, but some you can join anytime. You might want to check out local farms to see if they have the fruits and vegetables that you need and if they have a farm-sharing program.

If not, you can find local farmer's markets online and see what fruits and vegetables you can find there. It's best to look at the organic section even here, because some farmers include store bought produce to sell more variety.

If you cannot find any organic or local vegetables and fruits you can still do the detox, but using organic vegetables and fruits is the best choice.

Vitamins and Supplements

While you are on the detox, you will be drinking every meal and you will not eat any solid food. To insure that you get your required nutrition, you need to take a very high quality multivitamin supplement for the duration of the detox.

Many of the nutrients that your body requires to function will be coming from the multivitamin during the detox.

That is because the detox is going to be working on flushing all the nasty stuff out of your body. Taking a multivitamin will be giving your body the vitamins and minerals it needs to keep functioning while the detox gives your organs and cells a good flushing.

You Need a Multivitamin

As any nutritionist will tell you, you should really be taking a high quality multivitamin supplement each day anyway. A good multivitamin can help your body stay healthy. It also will help you maintain a healthy weight.

Your body knows what it needs and it serves these needs with cravings. If you are getting the nutrition you need, you will find it easier to stick to any eating plan you have.

Even if you eat a very healthy diet there are going to be times when you don't get enough of certain vitamins and minerals. Some minerals can't be gotten from commonly available foods and have to be taken in supplement form. Some vitamins and minerals are there in the foods that you eat, but not in the sufficient quantities to help you stay healthy.

So investing in a high quality multivitamin is going to benefit you even after you are done with the detox, as you begin a healthier lifestyle. Don't stop taking it just because the detox is over.

How to Choose a High Quality Multivitamin

Have you ever looked at the vitamin aisle at the local pharmacy or grocery store? There are hundreds of choices when it comes to multivitamins!

More so, if you go to a health food store or a specialty supplement store, there are even more choices. It can be extremely challenging to try to choose a good quality vitamin when there are so many on the market. According to their labels, every single one is the best! It can seem nearly impossible to choose.

However, there is one fool proof way to be sure that the vitamins you are buying is good quality. According to nutrition experts, if you want to buy a high quality vitamin it does not matter which one you buy as long as the vitamins come from food.

Synthetic Vitamins vs. Food Based Vitamins

Wait a minute, all vitamins do not come directly from food?

That sounds crazy, doesn't it?

It seems counterintuitive, but it can be true. In order to make vitamins cheaper to produce some companies use synthetic vitamins that are created in a lab.

Other vitamin companies break down actual food and extract the vitamins from it. Vitamins from food ingredients have the highest quality nutrition to help you stay healthy. That is the kind you want to buy.

Why Synthetic Vitamins Are Bad For Your Body

The human body is a complex organism. When the body breaks down food in order to get the vitamins and minerals out, it does not isolate each individual vitamin.

It uses those vitamins in pairs or groups to make it easier for different parts of the body to use those vitamins.

Vitamin C Isn't Just Vitamin C

As an example, take a look at Vitamin C. You need Vitamin C to stay healthy. It boosts the immune system. It keeps your cells healthy. It has been linked to cancer and stroke prevention, and even eye health.

Some food scientists say that Vitamin C can even help you live longer. Perhaps most important during your 3-day detox, Vitamin C helps your body absorb and process all of the other vitamins and minerals in your detox drinks

The base of Vitamin C is Ascorbic Acid, but the Vitamin C that is in food is a lot more than just Ascorbic Acid. Research shows that Vitamin C should be considered a complex of C vitamins, in a similar way to the Vitamin B Complex that is available. It also has trace amounts of other vitamins and minerals, called phytonutrients, that all work together with Vitamin C to make your body stronger.

Vitamin C that comes from food will be more complex, and have those tiny quantities of other vitamins and minerals that you need, but synthetic vitamins will have only Ascorbic Acid.

Ascorbic acid alone does not have nearly the benefits for your body provided by a natural form of Vitamin C.

Synthetic Vitamins Are a Waste in More Ways Than One

Synthetic vitamin and mineral supplements are created in the lab, but even scientists claim that they are "essentially" the same as those from food.

However, they are not identical chemically, and hence the body may not even recognize them as nutrients. Some of these manufactured supplements may even be seen as *toxins by the body.*

Science is only now beginning to understand phytonutrients and how they contribute to our health.

How can science possibly duplicate something it does not even understand?

Additionally, since synthetic vitamins do not have those paired up vitamins and minerals, the body does not know how to process them effectively.

Most of the time the body will not even process synthetic vitamins and they just end up getting washed out of the body with other wastes. Taking synthetic vitamins is a lot like flushing money down the drain.

Pick a Plant Based Multivitamin

When you are detoxing your body will need the best supplemental vitamins and minerals you can give it. So in order to give your body the support that it needs while you are on the 3-day detox look for a supplement that uses vitamins and minerals from food.

To find out if a vitamin is food based or synthetic check the back of the label carefully. Vitamins that are plant based will usually have a long list of vitamins that are in the multivitamin.

The label usually will say that the vitamins come from food.

If the label doesn't say where the vitamins come from a surefire way to tell is to look at the listing for Vitamin C. If the label says Vitamin C, then the supplement is plant based. If it is labeled Ascorbic Acid then you can be pretty confident that the vitamin is synthetic.

Organic Vitamins

If you are buying your supplements at a local natural foods store, you might wonder if a higher priced organic vitamin is worth the extra cost. Some foods are really not worth paying more for an organic label, but vitamins are worth paying more for.

The organic label on a multivitamin means that the ingredients in the supplement come from organic food, which is extremely beneficial to your health. A "raw" food label is a plus. Organic and raw foods have the highest levels of vitamins and minerals.

So if buying an organic vitamin is an option, you should spend more to get an organic or raw food multivitamin. Take this 3-day detox as an opportunity to not only lose weight but also start taking better care of your body.

Taking care of your body starts with investing in better quality food and supplements. When the detox is done, you will feel rejuvenated. Eating high quality organic food and taking a high quality multivitamin will keep you feeling great after the detox is over, and it will help you maintain your weight loss.

The next thing that you will need to make your 3-day detox a success is a good probiotic.

What Is a Probiotic?

Probiotics are certain forms of bacteria that are essential to your health. We think of bacteria as harmful, but some we actually need for our systems to work properly.

The term "probiotics" was coined to differentiate between the two. If you don't have enough probiotics in your body, or if the harmful bacteria are out of balance with the helpful bacteria, you can develop a lot of uncomfortable and unhealthy conditions.

Probiotics work with your body to keep it functioning the way it should.

Why You Need a Probiotic

Did you know that your body has both good bacteria and bad bacteria?

Good bacteria keep your body balanced and help your body prevent illnesses. Good bacteria prevent things like diarrhea, gas, bloating, infection, and many other illnesses and conditions. Bad bacteria can also cause skin problems like eczema and rashes.

You always have good bacteria and bad bacteria in your gut. But when the balance of those bacteria is out of whack it can cause some pretty serious problems.

This is another area science is only beginning to understand. Lots of things can cause an imbalance of bacteria in your body like:

- Getting sick

- Eating an unhealthy diet

- Taking certain medicines like antibiotics

- Eating too much sugar

- Stress

Taking a probiotic will introduce good and helpful bacteria back into your body. Those bacteria can restore the balance that you need to have in your gut in order to be healthy.

When you are doing the 3-day detox taking a probiotic will help get rid of the overabundance of negative bacteria and waste products that you are going to be flushing out of your body.

You can get some probiotic benefits from eating yogurt, because yogurt contains a very powerful and helpful probiotic agent. But, since you will not be eating any solid food on the 3-day detox you will need a probiotic supplement to bring your body into balance.

How to Choose a Probiotic

Choosing a probiotic supplement can be even more confusing than choosing a multivitamin.

In order to find a high quality probiotic you might need to go to a health food store or even order one on-line. A multitude of factors affect your choice of a quality supplement.

Live and Active Cultures

Have you ever noticed on a yogurt label the phrase "live and active cultures"?

That means that the bacteria in the yogurt are the kind that is good for you. The key thing you need to look for when choosing a probiotic is that the probiotic contains live and active cultures.

Probiotics are regulated as food, so there is no guarantee of quality. You must carefully read the labels to avoid buying a probiotic supplement that will not provide the healthy bacteria you need.

The probiotic supplement is required to give information on what it contains right on the label. Probiotics are made up of healthy bacteria, which are living organisms.

So, the bacteria need to be alive when you take them in order for them to do any good.

Viable Through the End of Shelf Life

A high quality probiotic will also say on the label that the bacteria are "Viable through the end of shelf life."

If the label doesn't say that it means that the bacteria aren't guaranteed to be alive when you take them.

Avoid any probiotic that says, "Viable at the time of manufacture" on the label. That means that the company only guarantees that the bacteria were alive when the supplement left the factory.

More Tips for Choosing a Probiotic

If you are still having trouble finding a good probiotic, you can use these tips to find one that will get your body back in balance and make the 3-day detox even more effective:

- Look for one with at least 20 different strains of bacteria. The more strains of bacteria the better.

- Look for one with one encapsulated pills, or other delayed rupture technology. That will keep the bacteria alive until you take it, and protect it from your stomach acids so that it arrives intact to your intestines.

- Check out the storage requirements. Some probiotic supplements need to be refrigerated but others merely require a cool dark place. Any probiotic supplement should be kept away from heat moisture.

- CFUs, or colony forming organisms, are the measure of how many good bacteria are included in your supplement, and you should be looking for 5 billion or above.

- Look for certification by a third party. Probiotics are not regulated as medicines, but as food, so choose a brand certified for quality by an independent organization.

Omega 3 Fatty Acids

The last supplement that you need to do the 3-day detox is an Omega 3 supplement. You are probably already familiar with Omega 3 fatty acids and the benefits they have for the body.

There are three main types of Omega 3 fatty acids. These are EPA, which helps with inflammation, DHA, which is essential for your brain's healthy functioning, and ALA, which your body can convert to either of the others.

Usually Omega 3 fatty acids are found in fish and fish oil, but they are also found in nuts and flax seeds. Omega 3 supplements are usually concentrated fish oil that is put into capsules.

Some people worry that these supplements can have an odiferous, fishy smell, but that usually only happens if they are low quality or old. Regardless, they have a number of healthy benefits for the body.

Lowering Triglycerides

Triglycerides are a type of unhealthy fat. When you consume excess calories, your body first converts them into triglycerides. When you have high triglyceride levels you are at a elevated risk of having a heart attack.

Taking an Omega 3 supplement can lower the triglycerides in your blood and lower your risk of heart attack.

Other Benefits of Omega 3 Fatty Acids

In addition to lowering your risk of a deadly heart attack Omega 3 fatty acids also:

- Lower your risk of developing dementia

- Help your memory

- Protect brain function and eyesight

- Promote healthy skin and nails

Omega 3 Fatty Acids and the 3-day Detox

Taking an Omega 3 fatty acid supplement during the 3-day detox will keep your brain functioning the way it should. Usually carbs and protein keep you alert, focused, and functioning.

Since you are going to be flushing out your body with a completely liquid diet for 3-days these fish oil supplements will make sure that you are alert and focused instead of fatigued and sleepy.

Detox Baths

Another element of the 3-day detox program is to take a detoxifying bath each day. The detox bath is an important part of the program and you shouldn't skip it. In order to prepare the detox bath you will need Epsom salts and Lavender essential oil.

What Epsom Salts Do

Most of the bath bombs and bath salts that are sold use Epsom salts as a base. Epsom salts are gentle on the skin but are great for detoxifying the skin.

Epsom salts gently exfoliate the skin and improve circulation. They pull all the toxins from the skin and body. Additionally, Epsom salts relieve bodily aches and pains, and this will be comforting to your body as it goes through the detox.

You may find that you like the relaxing detox bath and want to make it a regular part of your relaxation practice.

Epsom salts are inexpensive and you can find them at any pharmacy.

You can mix them with different flowers, herbs, or oils to make your bath aromatic as well as therapeutic.

Lavender Essential Oil

For this bath to be effective you need to use a Lavender essential oil that is 100% essential oil and not fragrance oil. Essential oils are extracted from the leaves and flowers of plants. They have many benefits.

Aromatherapy uses pure essential oils to help people relax and to treat medical conditions. Lavender essential oil is one of the gentlest essential oils. It is even used on babies to help them sleep and relax.

Lavender smells wonderful.

Adding Lavender essential oil to your bath will help you relax, improve your quality of sleep, and heal your skin. Lavender oil is often used to treat skin conditions like dry skin, eczema, rashes, burns, and acne.

Adding this essential oil to your bath water will make your skin soft and beautiful after the Epsom salts have pulled all the gross pollutants, dead skin and other harmful elements out of your body.

Substitutions

If you don't like the scent of Lavender essential oil you can use another gentle essential oil. Tea Tree essential oil is a great choice, as it has many of the same positive benefits of Lavender.

Just make sure that whatever oil you use is a pure essential oil and not a fragrance oil. Fragrance oils are synthetic and made to be used in perfumes and soaps. They have no healing benefits.

Some detox baths include apple cider vinegar, sea salt, baking soda, or ginger. You may decide you would like to try including these. They cause you to sweat, which aids the Epsom salts in drawing toxins out of your body.

The 3-day Detox Shopping List

Remember to get organic fruits and vegetables whenever possible for the best nutrition. You may get more of each item if you want, in case you need it, but the amount given is the minimum suggested amount to buy.

The list might look overwhelming. However, you will be given a choice of several drinks for each meal.

The following list is composed as if you were going to make all of them. Of course, in 3 days, you will only sample a few. So, here is where planning ahead comes in very handy.

Look ahead to Chapter 4, and see which drinks sound best to you. It will be a snap to stick to your liquid diet if you enjoy the drinks!

After picking out your tasty liquid meals, narrow the master list to a shopping list for those detox drinks you decided on. Once you have refined your list, stick to it.

You will thereby have an easier time sticking to your plan of completing the 3 day detox. Make sure that you also have a blender or juicer at home to make the drinks you will be drinking in place of actual meals.

Shopping List:

- 5 cups raspberries

- 6 cups blueberries

- 4 cups strawberries

- 3 cups cranberries

- 1 cup green grapes

- 5 mangos

- 3 pineapples

- 6 apples, 4 green, 2 red

- 8 bananas

- 4 pears

- 1 cup pitted cherries

- 2 oranges

- 10 lemons

- 10 limes

- 6 dates

- 10 cups of kale

- 5 cups romaine lettuce

- 2 cups red leafed lettuce

- 1 bunch broccoli

- 3 avocadoes

- 5 cucumbers

- 5 cup of spinach

- 18 stalks of celery

- 3 large tomatoes

- 2 red bell peppers

- 1 bundle of watercress

- 1 bundle cilantro

- 1 large root jicama

- 4 cloves of garlic

- 5 carrots

- 1 pint local honey, any variety

- 1 pint unsweetened cranberry juice

- 1 pint unsweetened pineapple juice

- 1 pint unsweetened lemon juice

- 2 liters of coconut water

- 3 cartons of almond milk

- 2 ounces (50 grams) of matcha green tea

- Cayenne pepper

- Ground flax seeds

- Whole flax seeds

- 1 fingers Turmeric

- Cinnamon

- Nutmeg

- Almond butter

- Coconut oil

- Green Tea

- Stevia natural sweetener

- 1 large ginger root

- Mint leaves

Bath ingredients:

- 2.5 cups of Epsom salts per bath

- Lavender essential oil (or your chosen substitute)+

How to Get Through the 3-day Detox

Even though you will feel rejuvenated after you are done with the detox and you will have lost a large amount of weight, it can be difficult to get through.

It is no fun not to eat for 3-days and only drink health drinks. You can expect to feel tired, cranky, and a little sick at times.

This is because the drinks and baths will be bringing all the toxins and sludge in your body to the surface and then flushing it away.

So it is totally normal to not feel at your best while you are going through the detox. That is why it is nearly essential to lay low for the 3-days of the plan. Of course, if you are normally an active person that much down time combined with not feeling well can be hard to take.

Instead of seeing the 3-day detox as something that you have to survive, though, you should look at it as a chance to have a mini-vacation to renew your spirit as well as your body.

Here are some fun ways make the weekend more restful, more interesting, and more rejuvenating:

- Turn your home into a home spa. Make homemade facemasks and other spa treatments to make you feel and look better.

- Pay a stylist to come to your house and give you a mani/pedi.

- Have an old fashioned sleepover with your best friend.

- Call friends on the phone instead of spending time chatting on Facebook.

- Skype with a faraway friend or family member.

- Read books you read as a child and remember how great it was to be a kid.

- Watch an entire season of your favorite show. Or, spend an entire day watching chick flicks.

- Work on crafts that you don't have time to do normally.

- Do some DIY home improvement projects

- Learn to meditate.

- Catch up on sleep

Tips To Help You Prepare for the Detox

Shopping in advance is a good way to prepare for completing the 3-day detox program.

But if you have never done the detox before there are some other ways that you can prepare too. Using these tips will make the entire 3-days run a lot more smoothly:

- Get a high quality blender. You are going to need it to blend all the drinks properly. You can buy a small blender very cheaply. A manual juicer, which is very inexpensive, might help with the citrus if you choose drinks containing it.

- Chop the kale. You already know that all the kale will be going into drinks, since there is no solid food eaten on this detox. If you don't chop the kale up into very fine pieces it can clump up in the drinks. Clumped kale is not appetizing at all. Chop all the kale into tiny pieces so that it will break up better in the blender when you are mixing the drinks.

- Drink your detox drinks at the same time each day. Your body's food schedule is going to be way off because of the detox. You may be starving long before you should have another drink, or you may not be hungry at all. Pick times that will be your mealtimes during the detox and stick to those times.

- Leave plenty of time to mix up the drinks. A few recipes call for frozen fruit. Freeze your fresh fruits for the best quality. The drinks contain a lot of ingredients that need to be washed, cut, and prepared. The citrus should be juiced, which is easy with a hand juicer. The liquids need to be measured. All of those steps take time. So start making the drinks about an hour before you want to drink them. If you finish preparation early you can put them in the refrigerator so that they nice and cold.

Chapter Three: Starting the Detox

Now you are ready to start the detox and start losing weight. Each day of the detox will be the same, so you don't have to worry about trying to keep track of any complicated eating plans.

This will start you on the road to healthy eating habits that will continue after the detox is over.

You will drink the same drinks each day of the weekend, so you can make up batches of one drink at a time and store the extra in the refrigerator.

This may help if you want to make preparing the drinks easier. Just don't store them for more than 3-days. If you have any leftover, throw it out when the detox is over.

Did You Enjoy 3 Day Rapid Weight Loss Detox?

Buy this book TODAY at:

TopFitnessAdvice.com/go/books

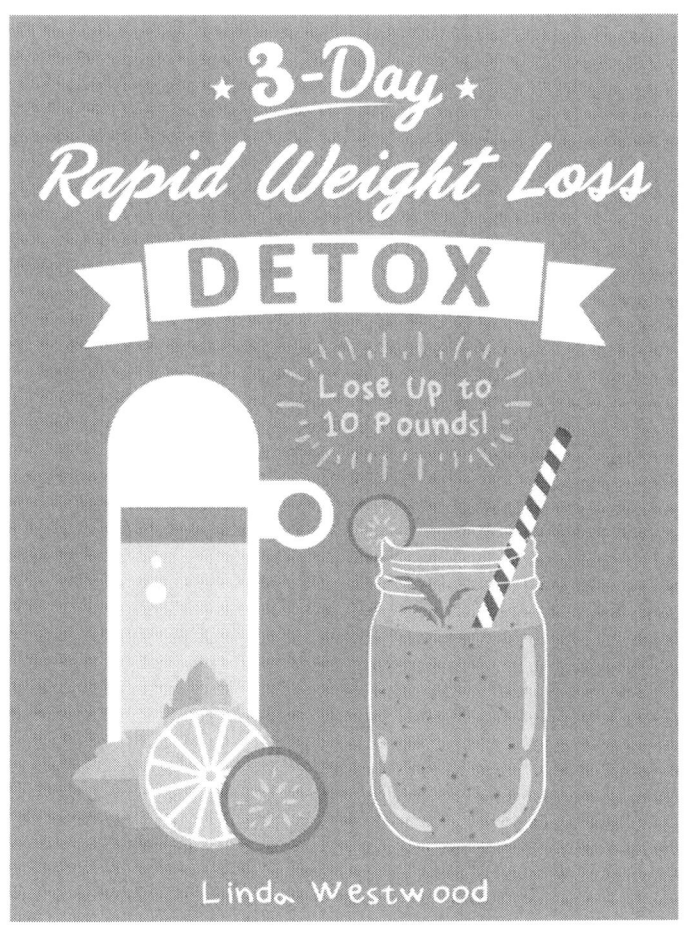

Sneak Peek
7 Day Juicing Cleanse & Detox for Weight Loss

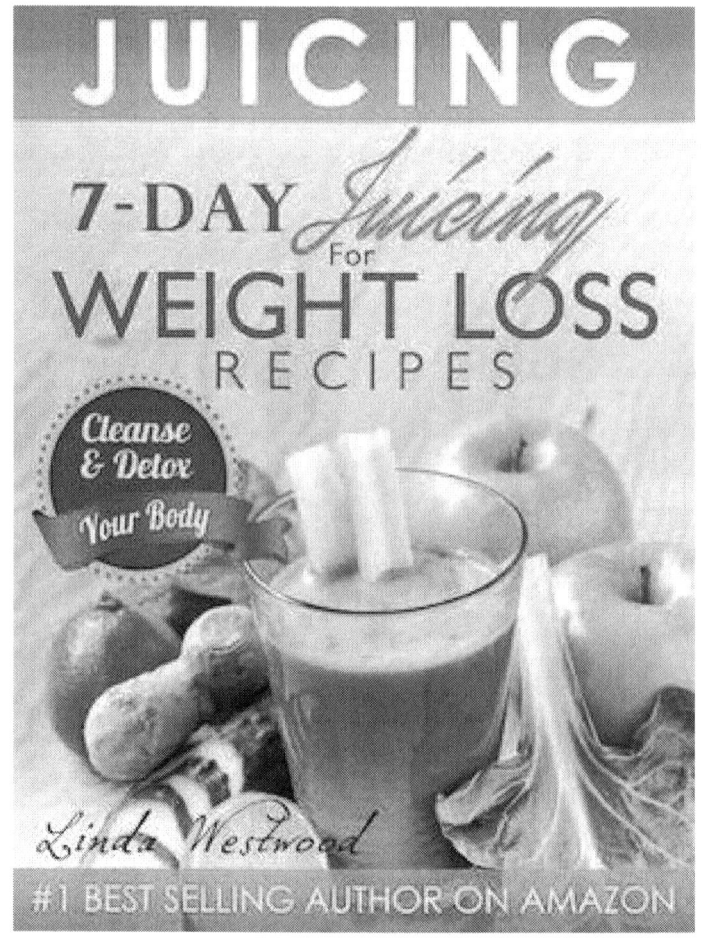

Buy this book TODAY at:

TopFitnessAdvice.com/go/books

Who is this book for?

Are you feeling tired and unhealthy lately?

Do you need to give your weight loss a *good* kick-start?

Do you ever wish you could just melt your belly fat *without even trying?*

Then this book is for you!

I am going to share with you one of the MOST effective juice fasts to completely cleanse your body from the inside out!

I have put it all together a full 7-day Weight Loss Juice plan, along with all the recipes that you need to lose up to 14 pounds in just 7 days!

The best part about this is that you don't even have to do any exercise!

You can be a complete beginner or someone who works out regularly, it doesn't matter!

If this sounds like it could help you, then keep reading…

What will this book teach you?

Inside, I will teach you this 7-day Weight Loss Juice plan that will not only boost your weight loss, but also clear both your mind and body!

You will feel the healthiest you have ever felt – have the most energy you have ever had – and the fat will be melting *effortlessly!*

How?

Because you're going to consume a very healthy juice plan that specifically plans out when your body needs certain nutrients – and then gives them to you in those juice recipes.

In this book, I give you the plan right in front of you that will change your life – all you have to do is follow it!

One of the most important things for you to realize when reading this book is that this juice fast *really does work!*

However…

For you to achieve *real success*, you HAVE to apply them to your life.

This is where most people fail – they read through the entire book but do nothing.

You MUST try your best to apply as you read through the book!

Chapter 1: What Is The 7-Day Weight Loss Juice?

Welcome to an exciting new chapter, both in this book and in your life.

The 7-Day Weight Loss Juice is an easy-to-follow, super-healthy, enjoyable and effective way to lose weight in just one week.

It will give you a huge boost of vitamins and other nutrients; all while the pounds rapidly drop off, leaving you in superb shape.

The 7-Day Weight Loss Juice is not a fad, or a 'miracle' cure. It is a scientifically sound, nutritionally beneficial, practical and fast acting way to shed unwanted weight at the same time as turbo-charging your health.

So what's the secret?

What is Juicing?

Juicing is a term that is becoming increasingly popular – and with good reason.

Quite simply, it means extracting the juice from ordinary fruits and vegetables and drinking it, with outstanding health and weight-loss benefits.

At its heart, juicing is a simple, highly effective way of extracting the most goodness from nature's best foods.

Essentially, you are gaining the intensely nutritive and delicious essences of fruits or vegetables, without chewing and crunching your way through the pounds and pounds of foods you would need to eat to gain the same benefits.

Easy on the digestion and excellent for rapid absorption, fresh juices are a totally natural gift to those who want to stay slim and healthy.

Don't mistake real fresh juice for the high-sugar stuff you get in cartons, let alone the 'juice drinks' with added sugar and heaven knows what else.

Real juice is made straight from the natural ingredients and is best drunk as soon as possible – no artificial additives, no sitting on supermarket shelves for weeks. Real juice is not a miracle cure but it is a wonder-food, one with infinite variations. Plus, when you learn about its amazing nutritional and weight loss potential of the best juices, then you will never look back.

Why is Juicing Good for Us?

Many people have never tried real juice. As you will discover, the fact that we don't make the most of the abundant fruit and vegetables on this planet is a large part of the reason that, according to the World Health Organization, as of 2008, 35% of adults aged 20 and over were overweight, and 11% were obese.

The bad news is that the problem is getting worse… but the really great news is that the solution is all around us.

It is hanging from every fruit tree, growing on bushes and springing up from the soil. It does not require exceptionally expensive equipment or specialized techniques. It just needs a desire to lose weight and a willingness to embrace the juicing lifestyle for just 7 days!

A real juice can be seen as an intense, delicious, flavoursome burst of nutrients, straight from the fruit or vegetables, in liquid form.

But what do they contain?

Well, it is no secret that fruit juices contain far more natural sugar than vegetable juices. While some natural sugar is fine, in order to promote weight loss it is best to keep proportions to 80% vegetable juice, 20% fruit juice.

Isn't Too Much Juice Unhealthy?

There is a misleading modern rumor in some circles that juicing is unhealthy and can even cause you to put on weight. Some even assert that it will lead to diabetes!

So, first of all, let's get a few things straight.

It is certainly true that the average fruit juice causes a rapid rise in blood sugar. This is not the same as when you take a large bite of chocolate, for example, due to the type of naturally occurring sugar in the fruit.

A healthy person would not be adversely affected as they can easily digest and absorb the fruit sugar. This means that the average healthy person will not get diabetes from drinking fruit juice.

Nor will you gain weight – obesity and diabetes are caused by unhealthy diets which mean your body cannot function as efficiently as it should; this simply does not apply to fresh juices.

However, some people suffer from certain conditions, which means it is inadvisable for them to drink fruit juices.

If you are even borderline diabetic, or suffering from candidiasis, or are prone to suffer from thrush, you should refrain from consuming fruit juices.

If you suspect that you may have a yeast infection in the digestive tract, or a low blood sugar level (hypoglycemia), or if you tend to put on weight very easily you need to get professional advice.

If in doubt, please do consult your doctor before embarking on the 7-Day Weight Loss Juice fast.

It should be stated at this point that some people have used low-calorie fasts to actually reverse their diabetes, but this should not be attempted without medical advice.

People who need to watch their sugar intake may still be able to juice, but should just stick to the vegetable juices.

Vegetable juicing, when done correctly, however, would not necessarily pose a medical problem in these cases.

There are so many green juice blends that you can try in the 7-Day Weight Loss Juice, all of them are bursting with nutrients and all of them taste delicious.

Plus green juices have many proven health benefits. You may have been told many times as a child to 'eat your greens' – this is just a palatable way of drinking them and getting an intense hit of their natural goodness.

Fresh green juices such as the ones described in this book may go a long way to improve your blood and health condition.

Read on to learn more about some of the major nutrients contained in a dazzling array of fruit and vegetables.

Which Fruits and Vegetables are Best?

Whatever the juice, provided it comes from fresh, natural produce, it is likely to be bursting with vitamins.

Here are some of the essential nutrients found in fruits and vegetables and their richest natural sources:

Vitamin A

Essential for cell reproduction, stimulating immunity and hormone formation. Supports vision, promotes bone growth, aids tooth development and supports healthy skin, hair, and mucous membranes.

Fruits: Grapefruit, Guava, Mango, Melon, Papaya, Passion fruit, Tomatoes, Watermelon.

Vegetables: Bok Choy, Broccoli, Brussels Sprouts, Butternut Squash, Carrots, Chinese Broccoli and Cabbage, Kale, Leeks, Peas, Pumpkin, Spinach, Squash, Sweet Potato, Swiss Chard.

Vitamin B1/Thiamine

Important for energy production and essential for a healthy heart, muscles, and nervous system.

Vegetables: Asparagus, Brussels Sprouts, Butternut Squash, Green Beans, Lima Beans, Okra, Parsnips, Peas, Potatoes, Spirulina, Sweetcorn, Sweet Potato.

Fruits: Avocado, Breadfruit, Custard Apple, Dates, Grapes, Grapefruit, Guava, Loganberries, Mango, Orange, Pineapple, Pomegranate, and Watermelon.

Vitamin B2/ Riboflavin

Promotes growth, reproduction and red blood cell production, as well as the efficient processing of carbohydrates.

Vegetables: Artichoke, Asparagus, Bok Choy, Brussels Sprouts, Chinese Broccoli, Green Beans, Lima Beans, Mushrooms, Peas, Pumpkin, Spirulina, Squash, Sweet Potato, Swiss Chard.

Fruits: Avocado, Banana, Custard Apple, Dates, Grapes, Lychee, Mango, Mulberries, Passion Fruit, Pomegranate, Prickly Pear.

Vitamin B3/Niacin

Powerfully aids the functioning of the digestive system, skin, and nerves, plus it helps convert food to energy.

Vegetables: Artichoke, Butternut Squash, Mushrooms, Okra, Parsnip, Peas, Potatoes, Pumpkin, Spirulina, Spaghetti Squash, Sweetcorn, Sweet Potato, Winter Squash.

Fruits: Avocado, Breadfruit, Custard Apple, Dates, Guava, Loganberries, Lychee, Mango, Nectarine, Passion Fruit, Peach.

Vitamin B5/Pantothenic Acid

Pantothenic acid is vital, helping us metabolise of food, form hormones and bolster our good cholesterol.

Vegetables: Broccoli, Brussels Sprouts, Butternut Squash, Green Beans, Mushrooms, Okra, Parsnip, Potatoes, Pumpkin, Spirulina, Spaghetti Squash, Squash, Sweetcorn, Sweet Potato.

Fruits: Avocado, Blackcurrants, Breadfruit, Custard Apple, Dates, Gooseberries, Grapefruit, Guava, Pomegranate, Raspberries, Star fruit, Watermelon.

Vitamin B6/Pyridoxine

B6 assists with the creation of antibodies in the immune system. It maintains nerve function, protein action and helps form red blood cells.

Vegetables: Bok Choy, Broccoli, Brussels Sprouts, Butternut Squash, Celeriac, Green Beans, Green Pepper, Kale, Lima Beans, Okra, Peas, Potatoes, Spirulina, Spaghetti Squash, Squash, Sweetcorn, Sweet Potato, Taro root.

Fruits: Avocado, Banana, Breadfruit, Custard Apple, Dates, Gooseberries, Grapes, Guava, Lychee, Mango, Passion Fruit, Pineapple, Pomegranate, Watermelon.

Vitamin B9/Folate

Folate occurs naturally in fresh foods (folic acid is synthetic and found in supplements). Folate is used to produce red blood cells, create DNA and support the nervous system.

It is essential for embryonic development, so it is especially important for pregnant women.

Vegetables: Artichoke, Asparagus, Beetroot, Bok Choy, Broccoli, Brussels Sprouts, Chinese Broccoli and Cabbage, Green Beans, Lima Beans, Okra, Parsnip, Peas, Potatoes, Spinach, Spirulina, Squash.

Fruits: Avocado, Blackberries, Breadfruit, Custard Apple, Dates, Guava, Loganberries, Lychee, Mango, Orange, Papaya, Passion fruit, Pineapple, Pomegranate, Raspberries, Strawberries.

Vitamin C

Vitamin C is an enormously important vitamin. It is an antioxidant, protecting cells against free radicals, which may contribute to cardiovascular disease and cancer. Vitamin C also has antiviral properties.

Vegetables: Bok Choy, Broccoli, Brussels Sprouts, Butternut Squash, Green Pepper, Kale, Swiss Chard.

Fruits: Blackcurrants, Breadfruit, Grapefruit, Guava, Kiwi, Lychee, Mango, Mulberries, Orange, Papaya, Passion fruit, Pineapple, Strawberries.

Vitamin D

Vitamin D is primarily obtained when the body manufactures it after being exposed to sunshine. It promotes absorption of calcium and magnesium, which are essential for healthy teeth and bones.

Vegetables: Mushrooms.

Vitamin E

Vitamin E is another antioxidant, protecting the body from oxidative damage. It helps form red blood cells and maximizes the benefits of vitamin K. It can also help heal minor wounds.

Vegetables: Butternut Squash, Parsnip, Potatoes, Pumpkin, Spirulina, Swiss chard, Taro.

Fruits: Avocado, Blackberries, Blackcurrants, Blueberries, Breadfruit, Cranberries, Guava, Kiwi, Loganberries,

Mango, Mulberries, Nectarine, Papaya, Peach, Pomegranate, Raspberries.

Vitamin K

Vitamin K is vital to blood clotting, regulating blood calcium levels and maintaining bone health.

Vegetables: Alfalfa (sprouted), Artichoke, Asparagus, Bok Choy, Broccoli, Brussels Sprouts, Cabbage, Carrots, Cauliflower, Celery, Chinese Broccoli, Cucumber, Kale, Leeks, Okra, Peas, Spinach, Spirulina, Squash, Swiss Chard.

Fruits: Avocado, Blackberries, Blueberries, Cranberries, Grapes, Kiwi, Loganberries, Mango, Mulberries, Pear, Plum, Pomegranate, Raspberries, and Tomatoes.

So there you have it – everyday, delicious fruits and vegetables containing an Aladdin's cave of vital nutrients. But we already knew that deep down.

What juicing does is help deliver these nutrients freshly, in substantial quantities and in easily digestible form. High doses of nutrients, relative low amounts of calories, especially in the vegetable juices which naturally contain less sugar.

But why not just eat fruit and veg, you may ask?

Why bother to juice everything in the first place?

The truth is simple, as it so often is.

Can you imagine trying to munch through six large kale leaves, two carrots, an apple, a handful of spirulina, a whole cucumber and half a lime – just for breakfast?

You would have a huge hit of vitamins, but it would take ages, you would also probably get indigestion… and feel pretty sick too.

Juicing the ingredients by putting them into a juicing machine ensures that you benefit from all of the nutrients, with none of the downsides.

But what about all that fiber – isn't that really good for you?

Yes!

But when you juice fruit and vegetable – *a lot of fiber is still there!*

Just to be clear, there are two types of fiber in fruit and vegetables – soluble and insoluble fiber:

Soluble Fiber

Soluble fiber is absorbent, much like a sponge. It enhances good bacterial growth, supports digestive health, regulates blood sugar control, lowers blood cholesterol and goes a long way towards giving you that full feeling.

Happily, juices – especially those with passion fruit, avocado, onions, apples and strawberries, amongst others - contain plenty of soluble fiber.

Insoluble Fiber

Insoluble fiber brushes the intestine, speeds up the digestion of food, adds bulk to the stool and keeps you 'regular'. Some of this is removed in juicing although it is still present in smaller amounts.

Also, some people choose to add a little pulp to their juice to bulk it up with natural fiber, others prefer just the purest liquid to ensure the best absorption of nutrients - the choice is yours!

7 Days to a Super New You

So, why does this juicing diet last 7 days?

There is no real mystery to this – we have simply discovered that this is the optimum time to fully reboot your system and let those incredible nutrients take effect.

It is long enough to let the vitamins flood through you and have a significant impact, to rid yourself of toxins and refresh your whole being from the inside out. At the same time, 7 days is a short enough time period to be sustainable, practical and enjoyable while being highly effective.

In just 7 days you can lose up to 14lbs, improve the condition of your skin, your digestion, your immunity and turbo-charge your fitness potential.

At the most serious level, it will lower your risk of having a heart attack or stroke. It is a relatively short period of time, but one which can transform your health and leave you glowing with vitality.

Read on and discover how juicing can reap health benefits that you may have thought were beyond you... No such thing, thanks to the incredible liquid power of super-fresh fruit and vegetables.

Chapter 2: Why Juice To Lose Weight?

So here's the question – what can juicing *really* do for you? Can it really help you to lose weight?

The short answer is absolutely yes!

When you take the right approach to juicing, the weight really can melt away, for quick and lasting results. If you are new to juicing you may not realize the full, outstanding potential of a true juice diet.

But first things first – how exactly does the juice work such wonders for weight loss?

Why Juicing Leads to Weight Loss

There are a number of reasons why juicing leads to fantastic weight loss. Here are the main weight-busting benefits of this juicing diet:

- Freshly juiced vegetables yield high quantities of nutrients for remarkably few calories. Fruits are also packed with nutrients, although they contain natural sugar so their juice should be drunk in moderation. With an 80/20 veg to fruit juice balance, the calorie total remains low (although you never have to count) and you will have the optimum results for effective weight loss.

- Juicing super-charges your system with the nutrients outlined in Chapter 1. Within days you will find that your system is functioning better than ever and, crucially, your metabolism will be firing on all cylinders, which promotes faster weight loss.

- Freshly squeezed juice is largely made up of water, which is great news, since so are we! The human body is comprised of around 60% water. It is therefore extremely important for good health to remain properly hydrated. Our digestive system and metabolism is fuelled by water, so a liquid diet can really fast-track weight loss.

- Living on juice for 7 days means you are eliminating other dietary baddies that may be causing you to hold extra weight. Out goes any excess starch, sugar, alcohol and fat, in comes deliciously fresh nutrients, water and fiber. Your body will thank you for it by rapidly dropping the pounds.

- Another important point to consider is that 7 days of juicing is simple to do and easy to stick to. With a good juicer and readily accessible vegetables and fruit to pummel into power juice, you can have a relaxing and enjoyable week. Far easier than cooking up complicated and expensive recipes every day, so there's nothing to prevent total success…

- … which means that when it comes to fast, safe, effective weight loss, juicing is good news all round!

Total Detox Through Juicing

The good news only gets better. Not only does juicing help you lose weight in a very healthy but fast way, it also helps you rid your body of nasty toxins, cleaning your system from the inside out.

The truly great thing about vegetables and fruits is that they are bursting with all kind of goodies that we often overlook in our regular diet.

Detoxing is not just about feeling better from all the things you are not eating and drinking, i.e. caffeine, alcohol, additives and so on, although this is obviously important.

It is also very much about the things you are putting into your body that work brilliantly to cleanse your system.

Here are just a few of the many natural ingredients that detox your system fabulously:

- Lemon juice is well-known as a detoxifying juice, one which gets your metabolism going, so a splash of this is always a good thing - it can also add 'zing' to some of the green juices.

- Strong colors bode well in fruit and veg, especially dark green in vegetables. Kale is full of powerful phytochemicals, while the chlorophyll in spinach is a first-class blood cleanser.

- Spirulina is a type of micro-algae and it is an ultra-healing detoxifying agent, so look out for recipes with a touch of this natural beauty.

- The natural superfood chlorella has detox properties, which help to eliminate mercury and other toxins.

- Beetroot is naturally full of antioxidants, plus nitrates, which allow more oxygen to flow in your blood and can improve performance in exercise.

- Ginger is packed with helpful compounds and has anti-inflammatory and antioxidant properties.

- Pomegranate is a very powerful antioxidant, even more so than green tea.

- Cucumber is superbly alkaline and soothing, so drink as much as you please to give you insides a treat.

This is just a short sample of the many detoxifying fruits, veg and plants you will enjoy on the 7-Day plan. All of the fresh ingredients that you juice will yield a wealth of natural goodies which will support or boost detoxification.

PLUS as they have naturally high water content, you will continually be flushing your system through with water.

Doesn't Detoxing Have Side Effects?

The short answer is yes, it certainly can have side effects, but this is essentially a good thing as it means the toxins are leaving your body.

We are living with more toxins than ever before in our busy, demanding modern lives. Chemicals in and on our food, in our drink, chemicals in skin creams, cosmetics and sprays, chemicals on our clothes… it is a veritable blizzard of toxins.

No wonder we are showing up with more allergies and intolerances – to stay healthy it is more important than ever to regularly detox.

The 7-Day Weight Loss Juice fast will do this brilliantly for you, which is why you may have the odd mild side effect.

When you begin to eat more natural foods that are superior in quality, in other words lots of fresh fruits and vegetables that are packed with nutrients, your body naturally responds to this vastly improved diet.

It sets about getting rid of all the inferior material, waste and tissues in order to make way for the new, superior materials. It then uses the new materials to create brand new, healthier tissues.

Unsurprisingly, with all this positive activity going on inside your body, you may notice changes, especially when it comes to the expulsion of toxins.

For instance, when you cease eating or drinking any stimulants, "fixes" that you may normally have every day like coffee or chocolate, you may experience headaches or migraines. This can be quite a common side effect, since it happens when your body smartly eliminates toxins like caffeine from your tissues and transports them in your bloodstream.

As these toxins travel on their way to their ultimate destination where they will be eliminated, they can cause mild pain or discomfort in the form of an aching joint, or headache and so forth.

You may experience other changes in your body during a detox of any kind. When you start taking in natural food that is of a much higher quality, it triggers the start of a regeneration process in the body.

Part of this process may incorporate a slowing of the heart rate, which you may feel translates as a form of lethargy or inertia.

If this does happen to you, do not worry and do not give up. Just remember that they are the evidence of an exciting internal regeneration process, which on average may take about 7 days up to a couple of weeks, depending on the level of toxicity in your body.

Use this time as a gift - take advantage of it as a period of rest, let your body recuperate and get ready to continue improving its own tissues. You are growing lots of new cells and literally becoming a new person!

Don't be surprised if you feel a little tired.

Just remember – it's working!

Have patience and rest assured that experiencing minor ailments is just a temporary state of affairs. Take heart by trying to embrace these inconveniences as proof that your body is changing for the better, moment by moment.

Knowledge is power and forewarned really is fore-armed – now you can relax during your detox knowing that you are not getting ill or going downhill, you are simply regenerating yourself.

In fact, with a few simple, pleasurable additions to your daily routine, you can maximize the effectiveness of your juice detox.

Max Your Juice Detox

If you are going to the effort of planning and carrying out a juice detox, you certainly want to do it as thoroughly as possible, right?

All the more reason to pick up a few more good habits, which will detox you faster and deeper, for more, lasting benefits.

Enjoy a Sauna

As you may be aware, our skin is our largest organ and responsible for the elimination of toxins to a huge extent. Most of us appreciate our skin but we should also learn to love our sweat.

Sweat, or perspiration if you prefer, is an amazing substance when you think about it – it contains scientifically measurable amounts of toxins that have been safely removed from the tissues.

It therefore absolutely makes sense to sweat more, especially when actively trying to detox!

For thousands of years there has existed a basic philosophy of striving to enhance human detoxification.

The Romans had their grand and decorous public baths, the Turkish relished their baths or hammams, the healthy Scandinavian had their saunas, and the Native American tribes had their sweat lodges.

In modern times, saunas can be found in gyms and health clubs, or even private homes.

We know that saunas are good for us because essentially and at a primal level, they *feel* good for us. We can feel the poisonous waste being drawn from our pores and the heat warming our lungs.

Nonetheless, for most people saunas are a very occasional treat. Why don't we spending more solid sweating time?

One reason may be accessibility, but also some people find the high temperatures uncomfortable. They should be aware that there are now more low temperature saunas.

A typical sauna is anywhere from 160 – 180°F. Most people cannot stay in such a small hot room for more than 15 minutes. The less common "thermal chambers" are set to around 100 – 120°F, so you can realistically stay there for much longer and sweat more.

But where you choose to go is not the point, the point is depuration.

Depuration is a fancy name for washing away toxins. The term is also used by fishmongers, when oysters, clams, etc., are rinsed with running water, to swill away toxins. The water essentially carries the toxins away.

Our sweat works in the same way.

Enjoy your time when you're in a sauna! Try doing a really good workout before you get in if you want to sweat more. Alternatively, go straight from the office and relax in the heat – the important thing is just to sweat!

Saunas can play a hugely important part of any detox regime. It will only boost your progress, so you have nothing to lose. If you have the time try doing it for 30 minutes daily, as part of your 7-Day Weight Loss Juice fast.

If that is too difficult, doing it once or twice during the week will also make a difference and make you feel good.

Just remember, sweating is extremely good for you. The more you sweat, the more pollutants are drawn out of your skin.

Learn to love depuration. However, make sure you remember to shower thoroughly afterwards, before you simply reabsorb them.

Dry Body Brushing

As the body's largest organ, the skin receives a third of all the blood circulated in the body. It follows that, when the blood is carrying toxins, they will be eliminated through the skin, a major organ of waste elimination.

So, taking care of this organ makes sense if you care about your health.

The benefits of dry skin brushing include:

Increasing the circulation to the skin, which is reported to reduce the appearance of cellulite. Cellulite is not just unsightly in appearance, it is lumpy-looking toxic material which has accumulated in the body's fat cells.

While there are some creams that claim to improve the appearance of cellulite, none of these expensive unguents has been widely proclaimed to be undeniably effective.

Dry body brushing on the other hand is relatively inexpensive – you just need a brush and a little time each day. The brushing helps shed dead skin cells and actively encourage the renewal of new skin cells.

This results in new skin, which looks smoother, brighter and clearer. As an added bonus, dry skin brushing may also help rid the body of annoying ingrown hairs.

However back to the main point – detox.

Dry skin brushing helps to greatly improve vascular blood circulation and lymphatic drainage. It releases toxins and promotes the discharge of metabolic waste. This means that after some dry brushing the body can function more effectively.

The nervous system benefits too as the process of running over the skin with a dry brush stimulates nerve endings in the skin – that's the lovely tingling feeling.

As if that were not enough, the act of dry skin brushing has been found to improve muscle tone and redistribute fat deposits more evenly, getting rid of that 'bumpy' appearance.

Furthermore, dry skin clogs pores and therefore helps your skin to absorb nutrients in a far more efficient manner.

For anyone who is serious some pleasant detox assistance, simply get into a routine of dry brushing every morning before your shower or bath.

It is very easy and you don't need to sign up to some exclusive spa to enjoy this health treat. All you need to do is buy a natural bristle brush (not one made from nylon or synthetic materials).

Make sure that it has a long handle, since that way you will be able to reach all areas of the body.

Here's exactly how you do it:

Set some time aside before you plan to have a bath or shower.

Take the brush and work in gentle circular, upward motions, followed by longer, smoother strokes.

When you brush, always begin at your ankles and work in upwards movements towards the heart. There is an excellent reason for this - the lymphatic fluid flows through the body towards the heart, so it's important that you move the brush in the same direction.

The only exception to this rule applies to your back. Brush firmly from the neck down to the lower back.

After your ankles, slowly move up to your calves and knee area, thighs, stomach, back and arms. Don't brush too hard over the softer and more sensitive skin around the chest and breasts, and make sure that you never brush over inflamed or broken skin, sunburn, or skin cancer.

After you have given your body a thorough brushing make sure that you do then have a shower to wash away the dead skin cells and released toxins.

If you would like to invigorate the skin even more and further stimulate your blood circulation, then alternate the temperature of the shower, turning the control from hot to cold as you wish.

After you have showered, do apply a lovely nourishing moisturizer. Keep it unfragranced and natural if you can (otherwise what was the point of the detox?).

Try pure cocoa butter, or coconut oil; argan oil is great for problem areas like scars or stretch marks. Then – your skincare work is done. A little friction, washing, temperature change and hydration can work absolute wonders!

Keep doing it and you could considerably lower you levels of toxicity, which is good for your health in a wide variety of ways.

But if you are going to the trouble of juicing, along with saunas and a bit of dry skin brushing, what exactly is there to gain from a juice detox plan?

The Benefits of a Good Juice Detox

There are many reasons why you will look and feel amazing after detoxing. A proper juice detoxification program is the health gift that just keeps on giving!

With this 7-Day Weight Loss Juice you will:

1. Enjoy a Great Energy Boost

The vast majority of people feel far more energetic after they have been on a really good juice cleanse diet. So many of the less healthy foods that we take in every day clog up and hamper our systems.

This is an incredibly common modern problem and stopping the flow of sugar, trans fat, saturated fat, caffeine and alcohol and instead filling up with only what our body needs and loves - including lots of that all-important water is - the best thing we can do for ourselves.

Plus it really is enjoyable to feel zestful and full of energy. Juicing lovers say that it is a wonderful feeling of the most natural, healthy, 'high on life' kind. No wonder more and more people are trying juicing for themselves!

2. Get Rid of Excess Waste

Detox allows the body to release excess waste, which is clearly the primary point of detoxing.

After an effective detox, the liver will be able to work more effectively and with added vigour, as will the kidneys and colon, which means your body will be able to purge itself of harmful toxins.

It is essential to keep the toxin load in your body as low as you can if you want to remain in the best health. High levels of toxins have been associated with all kinds of digestive and other disorders, or even severe illnesses such as cancer. A great juice detox like this one will reboot your toxin-elimination system extremely well.

3. Lose Weight, Naturally

We have looked at why juicing helps with weight loss in a natural, rapid, safe and effective way. However, looking beyond your 7 days of juicing pleasure, you are likely to want to enjoy continued good health.

That is why we use the term 'reboot' – it can be a new start and a brilliant way to change old habits.

Make the most of your 7-Day Weight Loss Juice experience by also using all that new-found energy to move around more – walk, dance, work-out and you'll feel fitter than ever and the weight will stay off.

4. Strengthen Your Immune System

With major organs like your liver and kidneys functioning better and with toxins being released, your body is better able to absorb critical nutrients.

One of the most important is Vitamin C, which is vital for your immunity. Also, dark green vegetables, ginger, oranges and lemons are among the natural foods which help to cleanse the lymphatic system.

Lymph is a colorless fluid, which contains the immune cells, which protect the body, so it is vital to your health that your lymphatic system functions properly.

5. See Your Skin Glow

As your body's largest organ, your skin is extremely important – it both supports and reflects your condition of health. A vital function of the skin is that it allows us to sweat and this is another way that we get rid of toxins.

You may wish to enjoy a sauna as part of your detoxifying regime, in order to sweat out those toxins as much as possible.

As a result of your 7-Day Weight Loss Juice, you are likely to notice your skin looking clearer, smoother and more glowing. Detoxes of this kind can also improve conditions like acne or eczema in some instances.

In fact, detoxifying may cause your skin to itch a little at first, but this will pass. The glow, however, will last for as long as you keep your fruit, veg and water intake at beneficial levels, which includes making them a key part of your daily diet after you stop juicing.

6. Change Your Dietary Ways

We all love a new start now and again. Rebooting your health with a detox can mean the start of a whole new era for the way your body looks and feels.

When you do something every day it can become somewhat automatic, even if it is harming your health and happiness. It can be incredibly hard to break those ties to sugar, alcohol, and fried foods and starch overloads.

A juice cleanse gives you permission to start afresh with your diet, in every sense. Rather than just 'give up bad foods', you are gaining delicious, nutritious, new habits that could easily last a lifetime. In fact you will feel so good, you will want them to!

7. Think with a Clear Mind

One of the favorite benefits reported by juicing fans is a much sharper, clearer mind.

This makes sense – think about how your mind feels after you eat a sugary piece of cake or too much pasta.

A sluggish body is never the best way to encourage lively thoughts. On the other hand, spring-cleaning your body will almost certainly encourage your mind to feel brighter too.

The removal of toxins and addition of nutrients really does boost every area of your health. Plus you should be brilliantly hydrated, which is far better for concentration.

8. Love Your Lustrous Hair

Every cell in our body is affected by our nutrition and that includes our hair.

The strand beyond our scalp is effectively dead, as all the growth is in the follicle, so keep it thriving with a detoxing regime. Some people say that after a juice cleanse they can feel the difference in their hair as it becomes softer, shinier and it grows quicker.

Lustrous hair is a good indication of top-to-toe health.

9. Lighten Up

This does not necessarily mean your mood, although that often happens too – it refers to that lovely light feeling that you have on the 7-Day Weight Loss Juice plan.

It makes complete sense – you are ridding your body of excess waste and toxins, your good hydration may have cured any constipation, you are not stuffing your body with heavy foods AND you are losing weight.

Little wonder you feel lighter!

The trick is not to panic and misinterpret the feeling as 'empty' or 'hungry' – you will be absorbing everything your body needs to thrive and no more. Enjoy the feeling of no longer being weighed down – the sky's the limit!

10. Look and Feel Younger

Aging is caused by various factors, including the damage done to the body by free radicals.

By boosting your intake of antioxidants, you are combatting the process that results in the visible signs of aging, such as wrinkles and coarser skin.

But the anti-aging benefits are not simply cosmetic - you can, of course, very directly affect your lifespan through your diet. We all now know that a diet, which consists of eating large quantities of fried food, is likely to result in a shortened lifespan for most people.

By the same token, a highly nutritious, low toxicity lifestyle that involves some regular physical activity is one that will not only result in you feeling your best, but also living longer.

11. Breathe Fresher

Bad breath can have several causes – but detoxing may really help.

Living without eating spicy, greasy foods, drinking alcohol or coffee (and of course not smoking) is bound to do your breath a real favor. However, there is more to it than that.

If you have bad digestion, or a sluggish colon, it may directly impact on the freshness of your breath.

Get everything moving nicely with a thorough detox and, after a possible couple of days when it may worsen due to toxins being expelled, your breath will noticeably benefit.

12. Feel a Profound Sense of Wellbeing

You should never underestimate the power of detoxing with juice. As well as the countless great things it will do for your body, it is also excellent for the mind and soul.

Many juicing fans report both greater energy and a profound sense of wellbeing, which has a positive impact on all other areas of their home, work and love lives. Feeling incredible – light, bright, hydrated, healthy, regular and perfectly nourished - can lead to great things.

In fact, it can ultimately lead to a far better life in every way... so there is no time to waste – let's get ready to juice!

Did You 7 Day Juicing Cleanse & Detox for Weight Loss?

Buy this book TODAY at:

TopFitnessAdvice.com/go/books

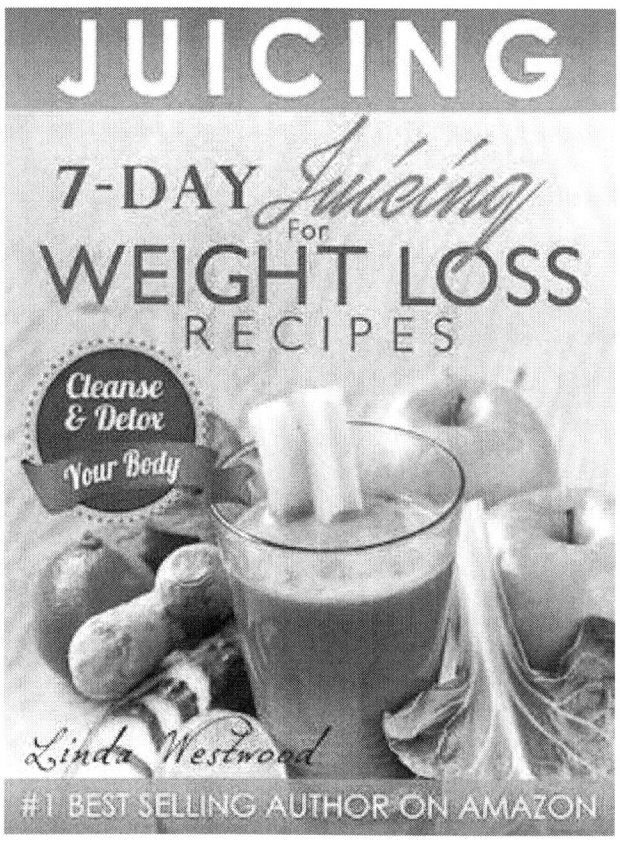

Sneak Peek
9 Day Weight Loss Smoothies to Cleanse, Detox and Lose Weight!

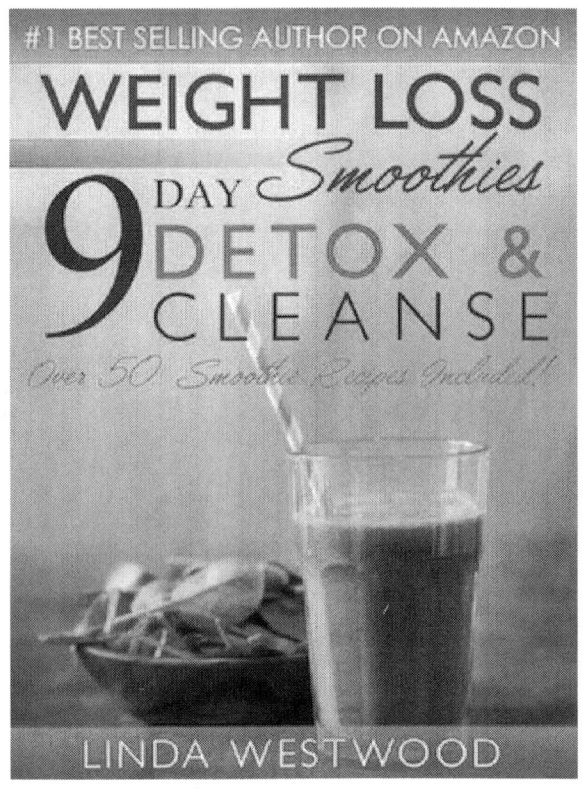

Buy this book TODAY at:

TopFitnessAdvice.com/go/books

Who is this book for?

Do you need a *strong* kick-start with your weight loss?

Are you constantly feeling tired and unhealthy throughout your day?

Do you just wish that your fat would just fall off *effortlessly?*

If you answered "Yes" to any of those questions – **this book is for you!**

I am going to share with you some of the best smoothies that will change your life!

I have put it all together in this awesome 9-Day Smoothie Cleanse plan that is set up for you to lose up to 17 pounds in just 9 days!

The best part about is that you don't even have to do any exercise!

You can be a complete beginner or someone who works out regularly, it doesn't matter!

If this sounds like it could help you, then keep reading…

What will this book teach you?

Inside, I will teach you one of the best 9-Day Smoothie Cleanses that will not only boost your weight loss, but also clear both your mind and body!

You will feel the healthiest you have ever felt – have the most energy you have ever had – and the fat will be melting *effortlessly!*

How?

Because you're going to consume a very healthy smoothie plan that specifically plans out when your body needs certain nutrients – and then gives them to you in those smoothie recipes.

In this book, I give you the plan right in front of you that will change your life – all you have to do is follow it!

One of the most important things for you to realize when reading this book is that this smoothie cleanse *really does work!*

However…

For you to achieve *real success*, you HAVE to apply this to your life.

This is where most people fail – they read through the entire book but do nothing.

You MUST try your best to apply as you read through the book!

Chapter One: What is the 9-Day Smoothie Cleanse?

This is going to be quite unlike any fast or cleanse that you have been on before.

Conventional wisdom holds that you need to eat a lot of fruits and vegetables but says that all fats, protein and dairy need to be excluded.

Whilst this does seem to make sense, it is not actually all that accurate.

Studies have indicated that the body can benefit from short periods of intermittent fasting. Fasting for two or three days, however, does not count as a short period.

If you are lactose intolerant, then you may benefit from cutting out dairy products, but there is no scientific reason to stop eating healthy fats and proteins.

In fact, you may even be harming your health by doing so, especially if you fast for prolonged periods of time.

The 9-Day Smoothie Cleanse allows you to enjoy the best of both worlds. Your gastro-intestinal track gets a bit of a break because the food is already mashed up and your whole body benefits because of the flood of high quality nutrients you are getting.

In one way, the cleanse is the same as the more conventional fasts – junk foods, highly processed foods and refined foods are off the menu.

You are also not allowed to consume anything that has refined sugar in it and cannot have coffee or normal tea.

It's not all doom and gloom for you java junkies though – you are allowed to drink green tea and this does have some caffeine in it.

It may not give you as much caffeine as coffee but it can still give you a healthy buzz because it is loaded with antioxidants.

You are going to replace them with food that is bursting with flavor. The advantage here is that the plan is designed so that you get maximum detox benefits without needing to starve yourself or having to rely on unsatisfying vegetable broth to help you get through the day.

Protein and healthy fats are an essential part of any eating plan. If your body does not get enough protein from the food you eat, it starts to use the protein stored in your muscles.

Fat, unfortunately, has the opposite effect – if you are not getting enough, the body will minimize its usage of fat and try to store any fat that it is receiving.

From this standpoint, it is difficult to see why anyone fasts at all. It is too much of a drastic measure, especially when you can get much better results by just doing the smoothie cleanse.

The key is in using quality ingredients in your smoothie and by mixing up the recipes a bit. Even though you have to have at least one smoothie a day, it need not always be the same recipe.

The proponents of fasts make it sound as though your body is completely inefficient when it comes to getting rid of waste. The truth is somewhat different – your body is busy detoxing itself right now.

Because of our typical modern lifestyles, this process may not be as efficient as it should be – we pile toxins into our bodies all the time.

A good analogy is a tennis player paying against one of those machines that automatically lobs the ball. Initially, the player manages quite well because the balls are not lobbed as fast.

After a while though, the balls keep coming faster and faster and our tennis player is getting more and more tired. He will get to a point where he gets overwhelmed unless someone steps in to help him.

To continue this analogy, the plan acts as an assistant for the player – reducing the speed of the ball machine and also helping the player by catching balls that he missed.

This plan basically works with your body to make the detoxification process more efficient by reducing the toxic load on the body and by providing your internal organs with the support that they need to function at full speed.

It is this process that helps you to lose up to 15 pounds in 9 days.

Chapter Two: Do Smoothies Really Work?

There has been a lot of press in the last few years about the benefits of drinking your nutrients in the form of smoothies and juices.

There are those that say that juicing is lot better and that it will help you to lose weight.

There are those who say that you have to eat "real" food and cannot "drink" your meals.

Others say that smoothies are too high in calories.

The truth lies in the middle ground – with smoothies, you are drinking your food but you are still getting all the fiber that you would have in the "real" food.

Most people actually start getting the right amounts of fiber for the first time in their lives because smoothies can be loaded with healthy foods and still taste good.

Smoothies do tend to have a lot of calories in them, but this is only if you make them incorrectly.

If, on the other hand, you follow the recipes in this book and you make them with the right ingredients, you will find that they are low-calorie recipes!

Remember that your body does need lots of calories a day to sustain it – the big problem with fad diets is that they reduce the caloric intake to such an extent that your body feels as though it is starving and holds onto any calories that it can.

That is one of the reasons why you often gain weight so soon after going on one of the fad diets.

Super Smoothie to the Rescue

This is where smoothies come in.

You add a whole fruit or veggie into a smoothie – and this will maintain its already high fiber content!

The blending does break down some of the fiber content but, on the whole, you are still getting your daily dose of fiber and the impact on blood sugar levels is not nearly as great as in the case of, say, store-bought fruit juice.

You will get enough of each type of fiber – soluble and insoluble.

Soluble fiber is absorbed into the blood stream and helps to mop up excess LDL cholesterol, keeping your heart healthier. Oats are a great source of soluble fiber and that is why you will see them in some of the recipes.

Insoluble fiber is just as important – it makes you feel fuller for longer and it is essential for the health of the good bacteria in our guts; it helps the food move as it should through the digestive tract and helps you stay regular.

Vegetables and fruits contain some insoluble fiber and some soluble fiber.

Let's face it - nature wants us to eat fruit and veggies whole.

Smoothies offer a bit of a compromise – you get adequate fiber and a shot of vitamins and minerals in quantities that are closer to what nature originally intended, in a convenient liquid form.

Your average smoothie contains about the same amount of food that you should be eating in terms of a healthy, natural diet.

The high levels of nutrients in the smoothies give your body what it needs to repair itself and so you will find that cravings go away.

The fresh ingredients in the smoothies are packed with antioxidants and so will help to fight the signs of aging and inflammation.

They will also help to flush toxins out of your system.

Additionally, you won't really feel as hungry as you used to because smoothies are very filling.

You can even tailor the types of smoothies that you drink so that you get the optimal benefits for your own personal condition – do you have a lot of problems with inflammation? Make sure you add plenty of nuts and seeds.

Need to get rid of gout? Celery is great at balancing the levels of uric acid in your system.

Smoothies taste good, are easy to prepare and fit in perfectly if you need to eat on the run.

They are the perfect way to lose weight – you just need to put the right ingredients in.

Chapter Three: Starting Up

Getting Your Head Around the Concept

Being mentally prepared is the key to success.

You are going to completely upend your diet and, initially at least, this is going to mean some adjustments.

Let's face it; you are going to be in for some discomfort – no change that is worthwhile is completely painless.

That said, the discomfort is not going to be as extreme as it would be if you were fasting – you are still getting all the food groups that you need.

For those coffee junkies out there, this will be a little tough but that is why we have included green tea as well.

You can drink up to 3 cups of green tea a day and, because of the caffeine content of the tea, caffeine withdrawal will not be as pronounced.

The tea should have no milk in it and should be sweetened with stevia or a little honey.

It is because of the symptoms of detoxing that I advise starting over a weekend.

By Monday or Tuesday morning you will be feeling a whole lot better – you just need to get through the first weekend.

The Epsom salts baths will also help to soothe the aches and pains and to speed up this initial detox period so that will help as well.

Any discomfort that you undergo is going to be short-lived anyway. Keep that in mind and you'll get through it.

Smoothies are Complete Meals

We are used to looking at smoothies as a nice side beverage. Consequently, we tend to look at a plan like this one and think that we are going to starve. What must be remembered is that smoothies are real meals.

With this plan, the smoothie recipes have been carefully chosen to provide a balanced meal.

You get enough fiber to help you feel full and the nutrients provided will give a smooth supply of energy without the spikes and crashes that make you feel ravenous.

Preparation of Food

Set aside some time to look out for good, healthy fruits and vegetables.

Go to you local farmer's market nice and early in the morning to get the best selection of fruits, vegetables and herbs.

It is best to try and get locally grown, organic produce. Also look for products like raw milk, kefir, farm butter, etc.

These usually taste a lot better than the store bought varieties and are a lot less likely to be laced with chemicals and preservatives.

If there is an organic farm nearby, find out whether or not they deliver vegetable/fruit boxes – many of the organic farms offer to deliver to your home or office and they make up a box of the fruits and vegetables that were ripe an ready for harvest.

Remember that organically grown produce may not look as perfect as the stuff that you find in the stores.

The upside is that it probably hasn't been subjected to a lengthy storage process and long cold-food chain. The imperfections are a sign that the produce is natural and good for you.

Don't be afraid to try different combinations – as you will see in the recipe section, there are a lot of different options – white beans in a smoothie, for example, make it creamier.

Kefir provides a great source of protein and calcium but also provides valuable probiotics as well.

Switching up the base fruit, the other fruits and the fats used is important because it gives you access to a much wider variety of nutrients.

Prepare as Much as Possible

If the morning is a mad rush for you, you might want to consider getting up 15 minutes earlier so that you have a bit more time.

You can, however, also cut back on the time needed to make your smoothies every morning as follows:

- *Keep all the necessary ingredients together* – set aside space in the kitchen cupboard to keep all of your smoothie spices, nuts and seeds together.

  You can even make little packs with the right amount of nuts, seeds and spices for one smoothie in each.

- *If you want to, you can chop up your fruit and vegetables the night before, put them in an airtight bag and freeze them.*

  This saves you having to put ice in the smoothie and saves time in the morning.

- *When you have to grind seeds, like with flaxseeds, it is best to do that just before you are ready to use them.*

  You can, however, measure out how much you need and get it ready in the grinder, or for those of us less technically inclined, in the mortar and pestle.

- Plan the day ahead and think about what smoothies you are going to make the night before you make them to ensure that you do have all the necessary ingredients before you start to prepare your smoothies.

What You Will Need

You need to start off with a good blender.

It doesn't have to have every bell and whistle, but get the best quality that you can afford.

Here are some things that you should consider:

- **How powerful the motor is** – You want a bit more of a powerful motor here because you will be chopping nuts and ice. Look for motors that are 500 watts and up.

- **How easy it is to wash** – Ideally, you should be able to disassemble the blade attachment and the actual jug of the blender from one another to be able to properly clean it out.

  This is pretty important – if the blender is tough to clean, it could end up being more trouble than it is worth to use it.

- **The strength of the jar** – I have used blenders with plastic jars and those with glass jars. In my experience, the glass one stands up better over time.

- **How many speeds it has** – With blending, you need only three settings – Pulse, and two different blending speed buttons.

  My blender has these settings – I usually only use the lowest speed. Occasionally, when a piece of fruit or vegetable is being stubborn, I use the pulse setting.

There are blenders out there that have several speed settings – this makes no difference, even my old, clapped out blender can blend a smoothie in less than a minute.

Tips for When You Are Making Your Smoothies

- Always put the fruits, veggies, nuts and fillers in first and ensure that there are no pieces bigger than a golf ball. This ensures a nice smooth result.

- Add in the liquids.

- Secure the lid and blitz for about half a minute.

- Check to see that everything got blended and make sure that there are no bits of fruit that got stuck under the blades.

- If you are adding any protein powders or spices, add them now.

- If you plan to add ice blocks, now is the time. Add them no more than two at a time, at most.

Check the manufacturer's manual ahead of time to ensure that your blender can handle ice. If you have added in frozen fruit, you can skip the ice. Consider adding frozen fruit or ice, especially when the weather is warm, it takes the smoothie up a notch if it is ice cold.

Check the consistency of the smoothie – if it is too thick, add more ice or water; if it is too thin, you can add more fruit or filler.

Chapter Four: Game Plan

How to Use this Book

The smoothie recipes in this book have been broken up into Breakfast, Lunch, Dinner and Mini-Smoothies, each with their own chapter.

Every day, replace your Breakfast, Lunch and Dinner with a smoothie from the appropriate section.

If you find that you are feeling hungry between meals, choose a mini-smoothie and have that.

In the mini-smoothie section I have also included smoothies that are good for specific health complaints like colds and flu, gout, etc.

All mini-smoothies can be converted, in need, to full smoothies – just check what you need to add in terms of the guidelines and go from there.

If you do convert it, it needs to count as a full meal.

The rules for this cleanse are simple – you must have three full smoothies a day, one of which must be a green one; you may have one mini-smoothie between meals if you are really hungry; you need to drink a minimum of 8 glasses of water and three cups of plain green tea a day (if you miss your coffee).

I recommend that you have your green smoothie for breakfast but you could switch it for lunch if you wanted to. Most of the smoothies can be switched to different times of day.

One word of caution though, be careful when it comes to switching out the evening ones – the breakfast and lunch smoothies have been designed to provide more energy than the dinner ones have.

If you decide to have a breakfast smoothie for dinner, make sure to have it at least 4-5 hours before bedtime.

Don't just dismiss a smoothie out of hand because of one ingredient – unless you have a specific allergy to it – try the smoothie first.

You'll be amazed at how different things taste when they've been whizzed together.

Naturally, not every item in every smoothie will appeal to everyone.

If that is the case, you can do some substitutions when it comes to ingredients, based on the principles that I share with you below.

You can also feel free to add extra herbs or spices to the existing recipes if that interests you. Do not, however, add extra nuts or seeds as these are very calorie dense.

Once you start getting the hang of how to put together a smoothie, you'll have fun experimenting.

The Basics a Smoothie Should Have for Weight Loss

There are tons of recipes available but basically they all come down to a few ingredients.

Here is what every smoothie should have in it:

- The base – this is going to be something like water, milk, or non-dairy milks

- A serving of fruit for flavor

- A source of high quality protein

- Some veggies

- A source of healthy fat

- Some sort of filler – to make the smoothie more filling. Oats is an easy one to use.

- Optional extras like sweeteners, etc.

The Base

The base is what will bind the other smoothie ingredients together and what makes it more drinkable.

Some people use a base of plain water; others use milk, yoghurt or dairy alternatives.

Coconut water and milk are just some of the alternatives that you can consider.

Experiment with different bases to see which ones you enjoy best and which ones work best for you.

The best news?

Low-fat is now being shown to be bad for you so use the full-fat versions instead.

As long as there is no added sugar in the milk you are using, it is good for you.

Almond Milk

Make Your Own Almond Milk

It is always better to make just enough to keep you going for a couple of days.

You will need:

- A blender

- Something to strain the milk with

- A container to keep the milk in – preferably airtight

- 500g almonds

- 3 cups of water for every cup of almonds used

- 5ml vanilla essence

Soak the almonds overnight in the water.

In the morning, whizz them up in the blender.

Strain out the almond meal and put to one side.

Mix in the vanilla essence and your milk is ready.

I add about a third of the almond milk back into the smoothie and keep the rest in a covered container in the refrigerator.

You will use about a cup or two of the milk per smoothie, depending on what other ingredients you are using as well and also depending on how thick you want the end result to be.

You can also use the milk as a healthy dairy alternative. Use as is or reduce the amount of water added in order to get a creamier result.

Bonus Tip: The almond milk makes a nourishing, cleansing skin mask.

Apply to skin while still damp and massage a little.

Leave on for about 10-15 minutes before rinsing off. Almond oil has long been used in cosmetics to nourish dry skin. The almond milk also exfoliates the skin, leaving it smoother and soothed.

What About Milk?

You can always, if you want to, use milk or yoghurt instead of almond milk.

The almond milk has got more nutrients and will give you more energy but it is not always a practical idea. If you are rushing, you can use normal milk or yoghurt to thicken the smoothie.

The milk, yoghurt or almond milk makes up the base and also the protein content for the smoothie. This will help to slow the absorption of glucose into the blood stream so do not skip this step.

If you are going to use milk, add in the same quantities that you would for almond milk.

If you are using yoghurt, the end result will be creamier and thicker so be sure to compensate by adding extra water.

Do use natural, unsweetened yoghurt and steer clear of any flavored yoghurt – the trick with the smoothies is to make them as healthy as possible and this means avoiding added sugar.

Another alternative is to use a milk product called Kefir.

Buy Kefir made from cow's milk NOT goat's milk.

The one from cow's milk is a lot subtler and you will not taste it in your smoothie. The goat's milk one tastes and smells awful, I don't care how good it is for you (my opinion).

If you have access to raw milk, you can use a little left over Kefir to start your own batch.

You just sterilize a jar and let it cool, add about 2 cups of milk and about ½ a cup of kefir.

Put it in a cool dark place for about three days until it resembles what you'd originally bought and then store it in the fridge. (It will stay okay for about a week or so once in the fridge).

Coconut Water or Milk?

It may sound odd to speak of adding coconut water or milk to a healthy smoothie – we have all been led to believe that coconut milk has a high fat content.

That is very true but it is also true that it is a high quality fat that our bodies can put to great use.

Coconut water has high levels of electrolytes and essential nutrients.

Coconut milk is extremely nourishing and tasty.

Make Your Own Coconut Milk

As with almond milk, make enough to last at most three days.

- 1 cup dried coconut – no sugar please

- 3 cups boiling water

- Pinch of salt

- Cheesecloth or tea towel to catch the bits

- Strainer

Place the coconut into the water and leave it to soak for at least 10-15 minutes.

Blend until as smooth as possible and then place in the tea towel/cheesecloth into the strainer over a bowl.

Let as much of the liquid drain through as possible and then squeeze out the rest.

Keep the bit left over to either add to smoothies as extra filling or use when baking.

Fruit is Served

Adding fruit into the smoothie is about more than just adding nutrients, it is also about adding flavor.

The fruit adds a touch of sweetness that makes the smoothie taste a whole lot better. (This allows you to sneak in those other veggies that you are not that keen on).

What you do want to be careful of is adding too much fruit because it has a lot of sugar in it.

You need to be careful about the G.I. of the fruit that you decide to add – you may add one serving of fruit with a high G.I. and one with a lower G.I.

Generally speaking, the sweeter the fruit, the higher the sugar content is.

You can add whatever fruit you like – it is pretty much all good for you, as long as you watch the serving size.

Try to stick to fruit that is in season – it not only tastes better but tends to be fresher and more nutritious as well.

If you are really battling to find good fresh fruit, frozen will also be okay.

Dried fruit is out completely – it has a lot of fiber but too much sugar that goes with it.

Fruit in the blender is easy – if you can eat the skin of the fruit, simply wash well, chop into quarters, remove the stone, if applicable, and throw into the blender.

You don't need to peel or core the piece of fruit.

In fact, adding in the skin is much better for you anyway. I also don't worry too much about coring the fruit or getting rid of the pips inside.

They really don't make that much of a difference anyway so you don't need to waste your time removing pips.

Do, however, remove fruit stones as these can damage your blender.

For this plan, you may add two servings of fruit at most.

Switch out the fruits that you use so that you get a variety of fruits and thus a variety of minerals.

If you want more variety, nothing is stopping you from adding 4 different half servings of fruit.

Freeze!

During summer, it is great to have a cold smoothie in the morning. Using frozen fruit can help make the smoothie taste good without you having to worry about diluting the flavor with ice.

If you are pressed for time in the morning, prepare your fruit the night before and freeze it so that it is ready the next morning.

Suitable Fruits for Smoothies

- **Berries** – fresh and frozen. It's a good idea to always have at least one tub of berries on standby in your freezer.

   That way, if you are rushed in the morning or were unable to get fresh fruit, you still have options.

   Berries are high in fiber and lower in natural sugars so they are a healthier option when it comes to blood sugar control. You could, for example, eat a whole tub of strawberries (no sugar added) without worrying unduly about spiking your blood sugar.

Blueberries are best in terms of anti-oxidant power so do have them at least once or twice a week if you are able to.

- **Bananas** – One of the stalwarts for a number of smoothie recipes, bananas are a great addition because of their sweet flavor and creamy texture.

  They contain a lot of magnesium and can help you to sleep because of this. They also help fill you up. You should not, however, put more than one banana in because they are so full of sugar.

  Bananas freeze rather well – do blend them while frozen though because they become very mushy when defrosted.

- **Pears and Apples** – Both fruits are great for making smoothies with. They add flavor, fiber and nutrients without adding too much sugar.

- **Pineapples** – Pineapples are the only dietary source of Bromelain, an enzyme that is known to aid the digestion, help alleviate inflammation and pain and assist in the treatment of arthritis and rheumatism.

  If you have an upset stomach, add pineapple to your smoothie – it will help.

- **Grapefruit and Lemons** – Grapefruit and lemons are great for weight loss. Try to use a non-dairy base if using these two fruits as the juice may curdle milk or yoghurt.

Grapefruits have been proven to be an effective weight loss tool – they stimulate the fat burning mechanisms within the body.

- **Coconut** – Coconut milk can provide a very creamy flavor to the smoothies and will help you to feel fuller. Alternatively, add pieces of fresh coconut, desiccated coconut or even coconut oil.

Coconut can boost the action of the liver and so is helpful in detoxification. In addition, the fruit is very high in nutrients and fiber.

- **Pomegranates** – These are one of nature's super foods. They are rich in nutrients and have been shown to have appetite-suppressing effects.

They have also proven useful in reducing the levels of LDL cholesterol in the blood and in helping the body detoxify.

- **Mangoes** – Mangoes are great in smoothies. Do restrict your intake to one a day though as they are high in natural sugars. That said, they are very high in Vitamin C and help create a creamier, sweeter smoothie.

Smoothies are ideal for mangoes – eating the fruit as is can be very messy and can cause sores to form around the mouth. Adding them to a smoothie solves both of these problems.

- **Papayas** – Papayas also have their share of natural sugars but are not as bad as bananas and mangoes. They also stimulate the digestive enzymes and thus help the digestive tract along.

  These fruits are also high in Vitamin C and taste great. Do make sure though that the papaya is properly ripe before eating it – if it is green it can cause a running stomach.

- **Passion Fruit** – The pulp inside is full of flavor and full of Vitamin C. These make great addition to both the taste and appearance of the smoothie.

  If you cannot find the fresh fruit, you can, in this instance use canned, as long as there is no added sugar or preservatives.

Bonus Tip: When it comes to the peels that you cannot eat, don't just throw them out. You can make yourself a quick beauty treatment.

Wash your face and then rub the inside of the banana or papaya peel all over. Leave for a few minutes before rinsing off and you'll have given your skin a boost.

If you are liking these tips so far, *you must* check out my 97 weight loss tips that are available to you right here!

If the link is still active, get it while you can, because I will be removing it soon (I can't keep giving away AWESOME secrets like these for free *forever*).

A Source of High Quality Protein

Protein is essential in this plan – it helps you to feel fuller for longer, helps in the building of lean muscle mass and revs up the metabolism.

You should eat a serving of protein with every meal. Your base will provide some protein content, but you need more than that.

Whilst it is tempting to turn to a protein powder, this is not the best idea if you want to lose weight. Rather stick to natural sources of protein such as nuts, seeds and yoghurt.

Alternatively, you can look to adding in more nuts or seeds to increase the protein content significantly. Chia seeds, for example, have very high protein content.

Tofu also provides a nutritious alternative to more traditional protein sources, especially if you are lactose intolerant or are allergic to nuts.

Get Your 5 Veggies A Day

The biggest benefit when it comes to smoothies though is that you can throw in just about anything when it comes to vegetables.

Because the ingredients are blended up, the taste is masked. This is great for those who are not fans of vegetables.

You can choose any vegetable as long as it can be eaten raw. Choose the freshest vegetables that you can find – if possible, grow your own.

All you want to have to do by way of preparing the vegetables is to scrub them clean and add them to the smoothie. With vegetables especially, most of the fiber is in the skins so if you peel them you will be missing out.

Do try to vary the types of vegetables that you use from day to day and try to get a good mix between different types of vegetables for maximum nutritional benefit.

If you really want to, you can steam the vegetables lightly before adding them. It is really best to eat them raw though.

Sprouts

When it comes to life giving nutrients, there is little that can compare to sprouted seeds.

It is well worth considering sprouting your own seeds as an additive to your smoothies, especially when you are eating green smoothies.

Sprouting is easy – all you need to do is to soak the seeds overnight, drain the water off and place them in a glass jar.

Place a piece of muslin over the opening of the jar and leave the sprouts in a dark, cool place.

Rinse with water every morning and evening. In a few days time, they'll be ready to eat. You want to eat them when the roots and stalks are about 1cm long.

Once you have harvested them you can store them in an air-tight container in the refrigerator. Stored in this manner they have a shelf-life of about a week.

Be meticulous about rinsing the sprouts properly – if you don't, they can attract mold and fungus.

If you detect a sour smell or there seems to be fungal growth, discard the sprouts. With practice though, that will seldom happen.

Once you really get the hang of it, you'll never be without sprouts again. To make it even easier, you can use sprouting trays in place of the bottle.

Also always be sure to buy seeds meant for sprouting. Seeds packed for planting are not suitable as they are usually chemically treated.

The Benefits of Sprouts

- Sprouts have hardly any calories and lots of fiber. They bulk out your smoothie without adding significant amounts of calories. Sprouts can be very filling foods.

- There flavor is quite different from that of the vegetable that they will grow into – it's a lot sweeter and a bit milder.

- They are a good source of nutrients and protein.

- They are alkalizing in the body – they help to reduce high levels of acid and thus contribute to the fight against inflammation.

- Eating them on a regular basis makes will help maintain your proper sodium balance and so also help to control problems with blood pressure.

- Sprouts contain digestive enzymes and also help to balance the blood sugar levels within our bodies.

- They increase detoxification by significant levels.

If you are liking these tips so far, *you must* check out my 97 weight loss tips that are available to you right here!

If the link is still active, get it while you can, because I will be removing it soon (I can't keep giving away AWESOME secrets like these for free *forever*).

What Sprouts to Use

- **Alfalfa** – Alfalfa is one of the most nutritious sprouts that you can grow. It is not by accident that it is so popular as cattle fodder and green compost.

  It has high protein content and is packed with vitamins and minerals. Added to your daily smoothie it will assist in detoxification, act as a tonic for the immune system and provide a seeming limitless supply of energy.

If you are only going to choose one plant to sprout, it should be alfalfa. The roots of the alfalfa plant go deep into the soil – much deeper than in other plants and this allows it access to more nutrients than most plants.

The sprouts have a slightly sweet taste.

- **Barley** – Barley is extremely nutritious. Barley water has been used for centuries to treat a variety of conditions from stomach ailments to diabetes.

   Sprouts added to your smoothie will help to soothe inflammation and irritation and alkalinize the blood. Barley is also good for reducing the symptoms of hay fever.

- **Fenugreek** – Fenugreek seeds are easy to sprout and have a more peppery flavor. Added to your smoothie, Fenugreek will help to soothe digestive upsets, balance blood sugar and cholesterol levels.

   It is also a great additive for detoxifying and will help to boost immunity. It has a bit of a peppery flavor.

- **Wheat grass** - is high in nutrients and a great aid in detoxification. It will help give you energy, rev up the metabolism and will provide valuable anti-oxidants.

It is particularly easy to grow at home and sprouting wheat grass is particularly rewarding. Wheat grass is sometimes sweet and sometimes a little bitter. I don't think that I would eat it on its own though.

These are very rewarding plants to sprout – they grow incredibly quickly.

- **Sunflower Seeds** – When it comes to plant proteins, sunflower greens take a lot to beat. They have the complete range of amino acids that the body requires.

  They provide support to the enzymes of the body and have amazing immune-boosting effects. These might not always sprout – it depends a lot on how old the seeds are – so don't be disappointed if they don't sprout.

- **Mustard and Radish Seeds** – These sprout really easily and add a bit of a peppery flavor. Also packed with nutrients, both of these greens will help to boost the immune system and help to detoxify the system.

  If you feel you have a bit of a cold coming on, mustard sprouts will clear it up in no time.

Other Vegetables to Include

When it comes to vegetables for your smoothies, the only "rule", as such, is to use the vegetables raw. That rules out vegetables such as potatoes and squashes but not too many others.

Wherever possible, leave the peel on – that is where a lot of the nutrients and fiber are. Scrub the vegetables well in need and simply chop them up roughly for inclusion in your smoothies.

If you are unsure about what vegetables to add, stick to vegetable staples like carrots, kale, etc. until you get the hang of things.

If you grow your own vegetables, or have a source at a farmers market, you can get vegetables that haven't been topped or tailed. This is great – you can add the greens into your smoothie as well for an extra boost.

Do use vegetables that are in season and as fresh as possible.

The beauty of the green smoothie is that it includes a wide range of things – the tops of carrots and beetroots, for example, can be just as healthy as the veggies themselves.

We usually throw them out because they don't taste as great. Blended into a smoothie, we barely taste them at all.

- **Kale** – Kale is similar in nutritional content to spinach but does not have the same high level of oxalates, making it the healthier choice for green smoothies.

The problem with oxalates is that they, if taken regularly, cause kidney stones. Cooking helps to rid the spinach of some of these oxalates. For better health, raw kale is the better bet.

- **Carrots** –Carrots are a wonderful vegetable – full of fiber, sweet tasting and chock-full of anti-oxidants.

Carrots make a great addition to any smoothie. Try using baby carrots for the ultimate in flavor and remember that you can also use the carrot greens in your smoothie as well.

- **Sea Vegetables** – Adding seaweed, etc. is a great way to source nutrients that we simply do not find in land vegetables.

The sulfated polysaccharides found in sea vegetables have anti-cancer, anti-thrombotic, anti-coagulant, anti-viral and anti-inflammatory properties.

You will also find them rich in various minerals such as zinc and copper, in quantities that are not present in land vegetables.

- **Cucumber** – Cucumber is a nice filler and has cooling properties. It does also have a range of nutrients but the skin is where the highest concentrations are.

The skin is high in silica and Vitamin E. Cucumbers will also contribute to your daily Vitamin C quota.

- **Beans, Peas and Legumes** – Raw green beans and peas are great additions to your smoothie. They provide loads of fiber and nutrients.

  You can also use chick-peas, beans or lentils, as long as they have been sprouted. If you just throw in plain lentils or dried beans, your body will not be able to digest them properly and they will cause stomach upsets.

  To remember what can be added into this category, it is easiest to think about how you would prepare the legumes normally – if they need to be soaked before cooking them, they need to be sprouted before you can add them to the smoothie.

- **Lettuce** – Lettuce is not known as being a powerhouse of nutrients but it can help with the detox process. Where it is truly valuable, however, is in your dinner smoothie. It can help relax you and facilitate sleep.

Hey There Herb!

To really increase the potency of your smoothies, you are going to be adding in some herbs as well. It is really better, as far as possible, to add in fresh herbs, but dry herbs will do at a push.

You will typically add in about 1/3 cup of fresh herbs or about a teaspoon of the dried herbs.

Don't ever use more than a teaspoon of the seeds at any one time and always ensure that the seeds are crushed just before adding to the smoothie.

As is the case with vegetable seeds, only use seeds that are specifically meant to be used for culinary purposes.

Seeds meant for planting are usually chemically treated and not safe for consumption.

Do remember that herbs, whilst all natural, can be quite potent. It is not advisable to add more than the quantities quoted above unless you are under the supervision of a qualified naturopath.

Herbs are really easy to grow and don't take up too much space so there really is not reason why you shouldn't at least try to grow your own.

If push comes to shove, you can grow herbs in a pot on a sunny windowsill.

Benefits of Herbs in Smoothies

Herbs have all sorts of benefits and it will really depend on the actual herb that you use. Typically, they all contain nutrients and assist in detoxification.

Herbs can be great for flavor as well.

I am going to list some of the more common herbs used in smoothies to aid weight loss but do keep in mind that this is not an exhaustive list.

Do yourself a favor and read up more on the subject – it is well worth looking into.

- **Basil** – You can use Sweet Basil if you like for a nicer flavor. If you are looking for perennial basil, Sacred Basil is a good bet. (It does grow into a fairly big bush though so be warned.)

  Basil has a myriad of benefits but primary amongst these is the ability to detoxify the system. Basil has anti-bacterial properties and is an excellent anti-stress remedy.

- **Celery** – Celery is a super herb when it comes to detoxification. It has strong diuretic properties.

  It helps clean infections out of the bladder and kidneys and helps to clear out uric acid in the tissues. (This helps to relieve symptoms of gout, rheumatism, arthritis, etc.). It acts as an anti-spasmodic, lowers blood pressure and is generally a good tonic for the system.

  Warning: If you are pregnant or suffer from any renal complaints, you should avoid using celery on a regular basis.

- **Cilantro** – Cilantro helps with digestion and boosts immunity. It also has a whole range of vitamins and minerals in it.

- **Cumin** – Fresh cumin leaves or flowers added to your smoothie will help with the detoxification process.

  If you are finding that you are uncomfortable during this process due to flatulence, a teaspoon of crushed cumin seeds in your smoothie will provide some relief. You need to either crush or chew cumin seeds to get the full benefits.

- **Dandelion** – If you have been putting your system under a lot of pressure due to over-indulgence, dandelion is a good option. It cleanses and supports the liver.

  It has diuretic properties but, unlike similar herbs, also as high levels of Potassium to replace that which is lost during the process. It also has diuretic properties.

- **Fennel** – Fennel has a licorice flavor that is quite pleasing. You can add it to both smoothies for the first three days to really jumpstart the detoxification process.

  It is a great additive if you have been overdoing the food and alcohol. Do give yourself a break of at least 3 days after using for three days though.

  Either use 1/3 cup of the fresh leaves and flowers or a teaspoon of crushed seeds. Be prepared, it is a strong diuretic.

- **Mint** – The primary benefit of mint is as a digestive aid. Mint will ease an upset stomach and also help you to feel more alert. It can also help in the first few days to alleviate the headaches commonly associated with detox.

- **Parsley** – Parsley's primary benefit is as a diuretic and detoxifier. It is also packed with vitamins and is useful in the treatment of gout, flatulence, feverishness and high blood pressure.

- **Stevia** – Stevia is the ideal herb for those with a sweet tooth. It is extremely sweet and can replace sugar. Depending on where the Stevia is from, a couple of leaves can replace about a cup of sugar.

  It is great for weight loss as it sweetens and satisfies cravings for sugar. It has a positive impact on blood sugar levels, blood cholesterol levels and blood pressure. It also helps fight tooth decay.

It is best to add only one or two herbs to your smoothie overall or you could risk overpowering the flavor that you have created. Do experiment with different flavors – the right herb can lift the flavor beautifully.

If you are liking these tips so far, *you must* check out my 97 weight loss tips that are available to you right here!

If the link is still active, get it while you can, because I will be removing it soon (I can't keep giving away AWESOME secrets like these for free *forever*).

Fat can help you lose weight!

Contrary to what we have been taught about fat, not all fat is bad for us. Your body needs fats to survive.

The trick is to eat the right kinds of fats – fats the body can use. Nuts and seeds contain monounsaturated fats and these have been linked to increased insulin sensitivity, better health and loss of body fat.

Fats added to your smoothie will give you essential nutrients and will help you to feel fuller. They also add a satisfying creamy texture to the smoothie and help you to feel full for longer.

Here are some fats you can add:

- **Nuts and Seeds** - We have already spoken about the benefits of almonds and some of the benefits of sunflower greens but here we are going to look at other nuts and seeds as well.

  Nuts and seeds contain these fats and are packed with nutrients – vitamins, essential minerals, fiber and protein.

  The problem is that most people can't just stop at a single serving and that is when the trouble starts.

  Adding nuts and seeds to your smoothie instead helps you overcome this issue, allowing you to get the benefits without overindulging. You don't need to add a lot either, about a handful is enough.

- **Coconut Oil** - The fat in coconuts has actually been proven to shift the body's fat-burning mechanisms up a notch or two.

  It is for this reason that people sometimes add coconut oil to their smoothies. (If adding oil, you need only add 1 tablespoon per smoothie to derive the benefits.) It also increases the satiety rating of whatever you eat meaning you can get away with eating less.

  Coconut oil is considered the healthiest of all the fats.

- **Avocados** – These are one of nature's wonder foods and everyone should be eating the. Delicious, packed with nutrients, monounsaturated fats and fiber, avocados make great additions to green smoothies.

  If you are only using half, leave the stone in the other half and place in the refrigerator. The stone keeps the other half from going brown.

- **Cream and Butter** – A tablespoon or two of either cream or butter adds a great tastes and is super healthy – especially if the animals have been grass-fed.

Nuts to Add to Smoothies

- **Walnuts** - Fight inflammation. Walnuts have more antioxidants than any other nuts and so are great at fighting of the free radicals that damages the cells in our body.

They also have the highest level of Omega-3 fatty acids and have particularly high levels of Manganese.

They reduce inflammation in the body overall and this, in turn, can help in the fight against painful conditions such as arthritis. Reduced inflammation also means a reduced chance of developing the so-called lifestyle diseases such as Heart Disease and Diabetes.

- **Almonds** – Almonds have more fiber and Vitamin E than any other nuts.

  A study published in the International Journal of Obesity found that the group who included almonds in their daily diet lost more weight overall than the group who didn't.

  Almonds offer powerful benefits in terms of protection against developing Diabetes. One study found that eating almonds daily decreased LDL Cholesterol levels and insulin resistance and consequently decreased the chances of disease.

  Almonds may also be good for the beneficial bacteria in your body. It is best if you can soak the almonds before use – overnight is ideal, if time permits.

- **Cashews** – Cashews shine when it comes to iron and zinc content. Iron is important in the fight against anemia and zinc is essential when it comes to your body's immunity against disease.

  Cashews also provide significant amounts of magnesium – an essential mineral that most of us are deficient in.

  Magnesium can help protect you against dementia and Alzheimer's and is necessary for good brain health.

- **Pecans** – Pecans are also rich in antioxidants and have been shown to not only reduce the level of LDL Cholesterol but also to help prevent plaque forming in the arteries.

  The high Vitamin E content could also form a protective function in the brain, reducing the chances of developing diseases such as Lou Gehrig's or slowing their progression.

- **Brazil Nuts** – When it comes to Selenium, Brazil nuts are super stars. You can get your total recommended daily allowance from just one nut.

  Selenium may help to protect you against developing some types of cancer. In some studies, selenium has been shown to slow the growth of cancer cells.

That said, you should not overdo it – getting too much Selenium can prove toxic to the body. Stick to one serving of Brazil nuts every other day to be on the safe side.

- **Macadamia Nuts** – Macadamias have a bad reputation for being fattening. They do have the most calories of all nuts but they also contain the highest levels of monounsaturated fats.

  These fats help to reduce LDL cholesterol levels and can help in the fight against high blood pressure. Mix into a smoothie that contains cocoa for a pretty close to perfect chocolate taste.

- **Pistachios** – Pistachios are one of the least calorie dense nut so if you are worried about the calorie content, they are ideal. Pistachios have high levels of Gamma-Tocopherol – a type of Vitamin E especially useful in fighting cancer.

  They also have a lot of potassium – vital for your central nervous system and the good heath of your musculature system.

  The B6 helps to improve mood and boosts immunity.

- **Hazelnuts** – Hazelnuts are rich in monounsaturated fats and Vitamin E making them heart healthy and very good for the skin.

Hazelnuts can help prevent deterioration of the eyes, and the development of dementia.

Seeds to Add to Smoothies

- **Chia Seeds** – These are said to be one of the Aztecs biggest secrets. They were especially prized for providing energy, improving stamina and for their able to make the eater feel satiated.

  Soak them in water overnight before adding to your smoothie and they become more like porridge than seeds.

  They are high in calcium, folate, iron, magnesium, soluble fiber and omega-3 fatty acids. They help to balance blood sugar and reduce inflammation in the body.

- **Hemp Seeds** – Hemp seeds do not have the same active ingredient found in marijuana so you cannot get high from eating them. They do, however, contain high levels of complete proteins and Omega-3 fatty acids.

- **Pumpkin Seeds** – These are rich in iron, B vitamins, magnesium, protein and zinc, as well as essential fatty acids.

  Most important for the dieter, however, is the high levels of tryptophan – the amino acid that is the precursor of serotonin. This helps to reduce anxiety overall and will help you feel better able to cope.

- **Sunflower Seeds** – Ever wonder why your parrot is so chirpy?

  It's because he eats plenty of sunflower seeds. Sunflower seeds are full of B vitamins, Vitamin E, protein and Omega-3's.

- **Flax Seeds** – These seeds made a name for themselves as the best plant source of omega-3 fatty acids. There is so much more to them than that though.

  They also have a lot of soluble fiber – great for helping you feel full and for reducing blood cholesterol levels.

  They also contain lots of lignans – a substance thought to protect against some types of cancer.

Spice it Up

Adding spices to your smoothies will not only make them taste better but will also allow you to enjoy greater health benefits as well.

Spices are added in smaller quantities – a little goes a long, long way.

You can experiment with the different spices you have at home but there are a few spices that you need to try in at least one or two of your smoothies.

Spices to Use in Your Smoothies

- **Cinnamon** - Cinnamon is a powerful antioxidant, fights inflammation and has been scientifically proven to reduce levels of triglycerides and cholesterol.

  That's impressive but not as impressive as its effects in terms of the regulation of blood sugar.
  Cinnamon has been proven to reduce fasting blood sugar in diabetics by anywhere from 10% to 29%. That's a lot! All you need is to add ½ teaspoon to each smoothie daily.

- **Turmeric** – Turmeric has been proven to be an effective anti-inflammatory agent throughout the body. It is used in traditional Ayurvedic medicine to treat upset stomachs and acid reflux.

  For the best effects, Turmeric should be taken with a meal that has some fat in it. (Making it perfect for your smoothies.) It is also best to take a few peppercorns at the same time to enhance the absorption of the curcumin – the active ingredient in turmeric.

  In addition, curcumin is a potent anti-oxidant and can help to slow down the aging process and also protect against lifestyle diseases and age-related diseases such as Alzheimer's and Dementia.

It is also showing promise in the reversal of the damage done by heart disease and in the fight against depression. You would add 2 tablespoons of Turmeric to your smoothie.

- **Cayenne Pepper** – Cayenne Pepper is a dieter's friend – the capsaicin content helps to boost fat-burning and to curb appetite.

  You need to add about ¼ teaspoon to your smoothie to benefit. Cayenne Pepper revs up the metabolism and helps to speed up the lymphatic system. Blood circulation is boosted and it helps to regulate blood pressure.

  It is anti-bacterial, anti-fungal, anti-viral and anti-inflammatory. You can substitute cayenne pepper for paprika in need.

- **Ginger** – Ginger is also great at soothing digestive upsets and at promoting the detoxification process. It has strong anti-inflammatory properties and may help reduce pain in the body.

- **Nutmeg** – Nutmeg imparts a nice flavor and has excellent anti-inflammatory properties. It is also said to be a potent aphrodisiac!

Fillers

If there is enough fiber in a smoothie, it is pretty filling. Sometimes though, it is good to add a bit extra filling to help make you fuller.

Choosing a healthy filler will further improve the benefits of the smoothie as a whole.

Here are some examples of fillers that you could add:

- **Oatmeal** – one of my favorites and I always use it raw. They help to balance high blood pressure, blood sugar levels, high cholesterol, and boost the immune system.

  They are packed with Vitamin B – vital for a healthy nervous system. They thus help beat stress. ½ to 1 cup of oats per smoothie will set you up with energy for the day ahead.

- **Oat Bran** – this is the outer kernel of the oat and is packed with fiber. It has a pleasant nutty flavor and is great if you need to boost your fiber intake. About a ¼ to ½ cup per smoothie is enough.

- **Cocoa Powder** – this helps to thicken the smoothie and is a great replacement for chocolate – in a banana smoothie, it makes it taste heavenly. Usually a couple of teaspoons will suffice.

- **Peanut Butter** – This is a multi-tasker of note. It can be a fat, a protein or a filler. 2 tablespoons is the maximum to add to a smoothie and do ensure that you get the sugar-free version.

- **Yoghurt, Avocado** – These all thicken the smoothie and act as good fillers.

Optional Extras

There are some optional extras that you might want to consider when making your smoothies – these can be used to enhance the flavor of the blend or to pack in more health benefits.

As with the other items, do try and get the best quality possible. Here are some optional extras to consider:

- **Sweeteners** – I would suggest that you try your blend before adding sweeteners.

  Normally the fruit will sweeten it up more than enough. If you are using almond milk with the recipe I gave, the vanilla essence helps to enhance the flavor as well. That said, some smoothies need a bit of sweetness.

  Do try to go for natural sweeteners like stevia or maybe raw honey. Raw honey is a great anti-bacterial so can be a good choice. You could also use xylitol if you have it.

  Steer clear of artificial sweeteners like aspartame and never use pure granulated sugar.

- **Salt** – A lot has been said about how we take in too much salt in general.

  On this plan, the opposite is more likely to be true – by eating all natural foods, you will not be getting much in the way of salt.

  Consider adding a pinch of salt to at least one of your smoothies every day. If you find that you start cramping, your body is asking you for more salt so increase your intake accordingly.

You can use good old table salt or Himalayan Salt according to taste.

- **Kelp powder or Spirulina** – Seaweed has a range of nutrients but it is not necessarily something that you have access to on a daily basis.

  Adding a teaspoon or two of these to your smoothies helps you to get the benefits whilst masking the taste – they do not taste that great at all.

What to Expect from a Detox and How to Deal with the Symptoms

What you need to remember is that we tend to follow unhealthy lifestyles. Sugar and caffeine are two of the most common stimulants consumed today and there is a very good reason for that – they are highly addictive. Ever noticed how difficult it is to stop at just one piece of chocolate or cake?

That's because sugar acts on the same pleasure center in the brain that drugs do. If you were to look at a picture of your brain on crack, and then a picture of your brain on sugar, it would look the same.

Caffeine is not quite as bad but is still addictive.

You are probably going to feel as though you are coming down with the flu and will find that your cravings increase initially.

The good news is that as you carry on going, you will find that the cravings also diminish and you will start to feel better and stronger.

The only way to get through though is to stick to the plan strictly.

Rest, drink enough water and do not cheat.

Here are some other common symptoms to expect:

- **Breakouts** – It has now been established that there is no link between the fat that you eat and acne. It has, however, been established that fluctuating blood sugar levels can have an impact on hormones and, consequently, on acne.

  During the first few days, your blood sugar is likely to fluctuate as your body gets used to the changes being made. This can cause your skin to breakout.
  This is normal and will not last long. As soon as your body adjusts, your skin will start to clear up again.

- **Flatulence and Bloating** – This is a very common symptom and is as a result of an increased fiber intake.

  You can try adding peppermint or fennel seeds into your smoothies to help with this. Again, this won't last long – once your body is used to the increased fiber intake, it will settle down again.

- **Constipation and/or Diarrhea** – Whilst not particularly present, this is again a reaction to the increased fiber intake. Again, it will only last a short while so do try to ride it out.

- **Brain Fog** – You are likely to feel as though you are in a bit of a stupor. This is generally because of withdrawal from caffeine and sugar.

  If this is a real problem for you, introduce a cup of green tea every morning and at lunch time – without milk or sugar.

  If this goes on for longer than 3 or 4 days, you need to re-evaluate what you are eating – you may not be getting enough calories, fat or protein overall.

- **Fatigue & Low Energy** – This is more a symptom of your body adjusting to the new way of doing things.

  Again, if this lasts more than 3 or 4 days, it is more likely a sign that you are not eating enough. Try to add an extra serving of protein to each meal and see if that helps.

- **Aches and Pains** – You are going to be surprised to hear this but there is very rarely a physical reason for developing aches and pains.

Chances are that they are all in your head – literally. You need to remember that your body is not keen on changing the status quo.

It is going to try all sorts of tricks to get you back to eating the way you were before. Think of these aches and pains as your body's way of throwing a temper tantrum. Again, this should only last a few days, until your body gets used to the new way of doing things.

- **Cravings That Won't Quit** – Your body can be compared to a toddler – it likes a set routine and will go to great lengths to get what it wants.

It can send out some pretty strong cravings. The trick to dealing with these is to make sure that you are getting the right amount daily in terms of calories.

You can also make adjustments to suit the palate – if your body is screaming for sugar, make sure that you have sweet fruit in your smoothie.

If it wants something salty, add a little table salt. The main thing is to ensure that you do follow the plan exactly.

Did You Enjoy The 9 Day Weight Loss Smoothies book?

Buy this book TODAY at:

TopFitnessAdvice.com/go/books

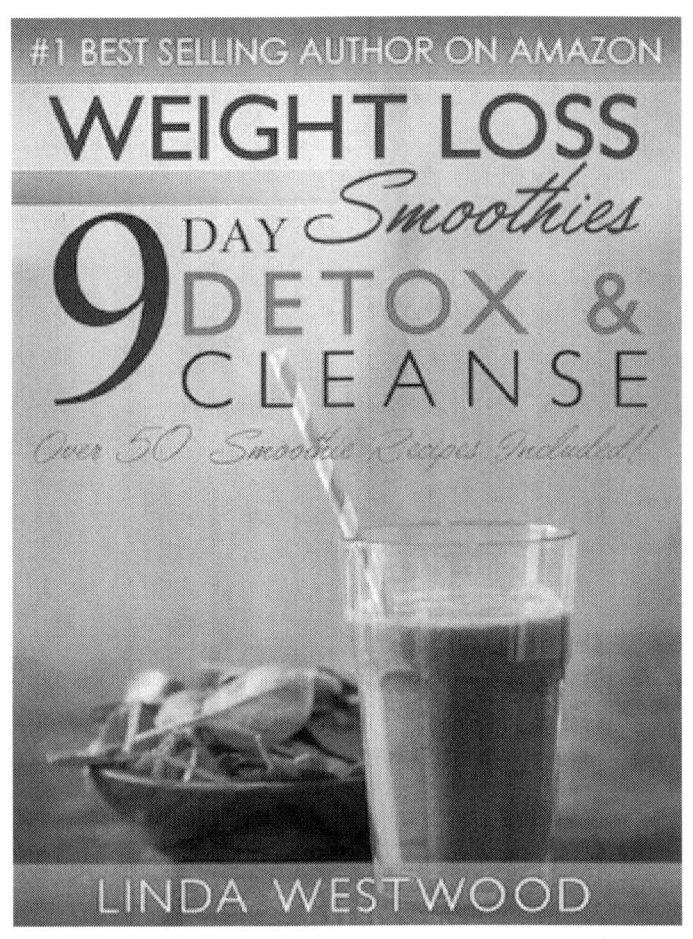

Sneak Peek
51 Quick & Simple Habits to Burn Belly Fat!

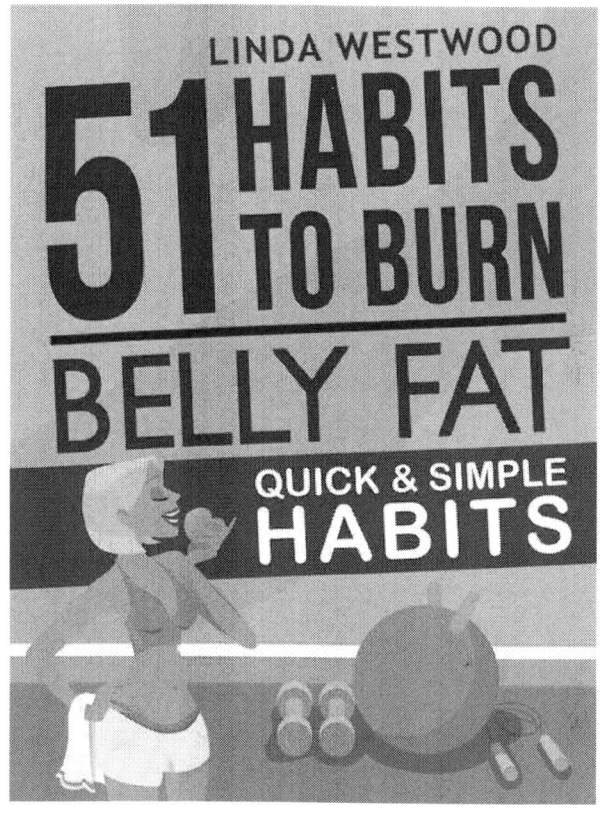

Buy this book TODAY at:

TopFitnessAdvice.com/go/books

Who is this book for?

Are you struggling to lose those last few pounds off your belly?

Are you sick and tired of endless crunches and sit-ups with NO results?

Do you ever wish you could just melt your belly fat *without even trying?*

Then this book is for you!

I am going to share with you some of the MOST effective habits that, when applied, will help YOU burn your belly fat without even trying – because they are going to be habits embedded into your life!

I have put it all together in this comprehensive book containing 51 of the most powerful habits that you can apply for maximum change in minimum time!

Since there is more to burning belly fat than exercise alone, or even diet alone, I have broken this book down into three separate sections for your benefit!

You can be a complete beginner or someone who works out regularly, it doesn't matter!

If this sounds like it could help you, then keep reading...

What will this book teach you?

Inside, I will teach you in great detail how you can start melting your belly fat without too much extra effort!

How?

Because you're going to learn which habits are the most powerful and effective at burning belly fat.

Once you learn what these are, and start applying them into your life, you will effortlessly begin seeing your belly trim up and become lean!

In this book, I give you 51 of some of the most powerful and effective belly fat burning habits that you can apply to your life.

One of the most important things for you to realize when reading this book is that the habits *really do work!*

However...

For you to achieve *real success* with these habits, you HAVE to apply them to your life *consistently.*

This is where most people fail – they try out a few habits and then just forget about them all, or even worse, read through the entire book but do nothing.

You MUST try your best to apply these habits as you read through the book!

Introduction

This book will give you the information that you need to start taking control of your health and losing belly fat right now.

If you haven't been able to lose weight before it's not because you don't have enough willpower, it's because you didn't have the right information.

How you eat, how you workout and how you live your life all impact your weight. Once you finish this book you'll know how to make better choices and live a healthier life forever.

Here's what you'll learn:

20 Eating Habits

The food that you eat is fuel for your body. These 20 healthy habits will teach you to eat food that is healthy and tastes good so that you will be able to lose fat and still not feel deprived.

Dieting doesn't help you lose weight, but changing the way that you eat and the way that you think about food will help you lose weight and keep it off forever.

20 Workout Habits

Working out doesn't have to be a chore. Changing your workout habits and finding exercises that you really enjoy will change the way that you view exercise.

Your body was made to move. Working out can be something that you enjoy when you change the way that you exercise to get the most out of your workouts.

Even if you have trouble working out at first you'll find that as you keep going it will get easier because the more you move your body the better your body will move.

11 Lifestyle Habits

Getting healthy means making some lifestyle changes. But, changing your lifestyle doesn't mean that you have to make sweeping or radical changes in order to see positive results.

Small changes in your lifestyle and way of thinking will add up to big results. Changing your lifestyle in healthy ways will not only help you lose weight it will also help you lower your stress level, increase your overall health, and make you happier for the rest of your life.

Give these changes a chance and you will be amazed at how you can transform your body and your life.

Powerful Eating Habits

Changing your relationship with food is the best way to lose fat and stay healthy for the rest of your life.

Do you know why diets don't work?

Diets don't work because they don't change the way that you view food. In order to lose weight and keep it off you need to change your entire approach to eating instead of just restricting what you eat.

You don't need to deprive yourself of food in order to lose weight or stay at a healthy weight. You need to eat the foods that will nourish and sustain your body instead of eating food that will hurt your body.

And don't be fooled into thinking that what you're eating isn't hurting your body.

Obesity numbers are at an all-time high. Heart disease, high cholesterol and other medical issues are also reaching epidemic proportions primarily because of the food that people are eating.

High carb, high sugar, and high fat foods will destroy your body over time and make you gain weight. Your body can't process refined sugar. It doesn't break down refined sugar and use it for fuel, so that sugar is converted into fat. Natural sugars are broken down by the body and converted into fuel. So just cutting out refined sugar and eating foods that contain natural sugar, like fruit, can make a huge difference in your health and have a big impact on your weight.

What you eat is more important that how much you eat. When you are eating healthy food that provides fuel for your body you don't need to deprive yourself of food in order to lose weight.

Starving yourself won't make you lose weight. Only changing the foods that you're eating can do that.

It can be difficult to change how you eat. Most people have a long list of excuses to rationalize why they can't eat healthy.

Some of the most common excuses people give for eating a terrible diet are:

- Healthy food isn't tasty.
- I can't cook.
- I'm too busy to cook for every meal and fast food is just easier.
- I'm on a budget.
- There's no point in cooking for just 1 or 2 people.

Do any of those excuses sound familiar?

But that's all they are – excuses.

There is no reason you can't eat healthy food and change your life.

These powerful eating habits will teach you how to build a new and healthy relationship with food that won't require you to be a gourmet chef, have unlimited funds to spend on food, or never have a tasty treat.

Eating Habit #1 – Cut Down On The Carbs

One of the easiest and most effective ways to lose belly fat is to cut carbs and change the carbs that you do eat.

Modern diets use a lot of carbs as fillers. Pasta, bread, rice and other carb heavy foods are staples that people at every meal. But those carbs are causing you to gain weight and can make it impossible to lose fat.

How Carbs Make You Fat

When you eat carbs, they are broken down by the body into glucose. When your blood has too much glucose in it, the body turns that glucose into fat and stores it for extra energy. But that fat builds up, and builds up more when you keep eating carbs and your body doesn't need the extra energy.

That's what makes you gain weight.

Pasta, bread and other foods made from refined flour are almost entirely made of starch, which is quickly converted to glucose and then is turned into fat.

Small amounts of fat are deposited into your liver for storage but the rest has nowhere to go so the body deposits it wherever there is room like your arms, your belly, your thighs and so on.

Healthy Carbs Vs. Unhealthy Carbs

Not all carbs are unhealthy.

Your body does need carbs to function effectively. Your brain also needs carbs in order to keep working. But you should be eating healthy carbs instead of unhealthy ones and eating only small amounts of them.

Healthy carbs come from natural sources like vegetables and some fruits. Fruits also contain natural sugar so they should be eaten in small amounts.

Eating healthy carbs will give you the energy that you need without causing weight gain. A combination of protein and healthy carbs will turn your body into a fat burning machine because your body will burn all that stored fat for energy.

Getting into the habit of eating healthy carbs instead of carbs from bread, rice or pasta will keep you healthy and help you lose fat.

Cutting carbs out of your diet can be tough, especially if you are on a tight budget. High carb foods are usually much cheaper than healthy fresh fruits and vegetables.

Here are some easy ways that you can start cutting carbs out of your diet without dramatically changing how you eat:

- Use lettuce instead of bread for a sandwich or burger. All you really need is a wrapper for your burger or sandwich so use lettuce instead of high carb bread.

- Eat more eggs. Eggs are a cheap source of protein that anyone can afford. Hard-boil some for quick and easy snacks.

- Swap pasta noodles for zoodles. You can make noodles from vegetables like zucchini so that you can still enjoy your favorite pasta dishes without high carb pasta.

Eating Habit #2 – Stop Drinking Soda

Soda is one of the worst things that you can put in your body. If you want to lose fat and be healthy you need to stop drinking it.

Regular soda is high in calories and has a massive amount of sugar.

Diet sodas are even worse, and studies have proven that the artificial sweeteners in diet soda can lead to weight gain. It can be hard to give up soda but you will feel better and lose weight if you stop drinking it.

Why Soda is the Worst Drink

There are lots of unhealthy drinks out there but soda is the worst because of the way that the high amounts of sugar and artificial sweeteners affect the body.

Eating or drinking a lot of sugar will wreak havoc on your body. Your body has to work even harder to break down the sugar and it will get stored in the body as fat.

The body uses insulin to break down sugar, so the more sugar you eat or drink the more insulin your body will produce. That causes too much insulin in the body. When the body has too much insulin it will make your blood sugar drop and can lead to poor concentration, fatigue, and other problems.

Diet soda is even worse. The artificial sweeteners used in diet soda have been linked to metabolic disorder and even to diabetes.

Healthy Alternatives to Soda

The best thing to drink is water. But if you just can't force yourself to drink plain water there are lots of ways that you can make water more appealing.

If you like the carbonation in sodas try drinking sparkling water.

You can add some cucumber slices or lemon juice to the sparkling water for a tasty and refreshing drink. Or you can mix a small amount of natural fruit juice with some sparkling water to create a fruit spritzer.

Herbal tea is another great alternative to soda because you can drink it hot or cold.

Most people drink soda because it's easy to find everywhere and it's usually pretty cheap.

Here are some easy ways to avoid falling into the trap of drinking soda just because it's what is available:

- Get a water bottle. Having a water bottle with you will ensure that you have a healthy drink with you no matter where you go.

- Bring a tea bag to restaurants. Most restaurants won't charge you for hot water so instead of ordering a soda, just ask for some hot water and have tea.

• Stash some water at the office and in your car. If you have water within reach you won't be tempted to get a soda from a vending machine or at the store.

Eating Habit #3 – Eat Vegetables With Every Meal

Remember when you were young and your parents told you to eat all your vegetables?

That's still good advice.

You should be eating probably double the amount of vegetables that you are eating every day. In fact, most of the carbs that you eat during the day should be coming from vegetables. You should be having at least one serving of vegetables with every meal, even breakfast.

Why Vegetables Are So Important

Vegetables contain the vitamins and minerals that your body needs to stay healthy and work efficiently.

They are low in calories and carbs and yet they are filling. Because they are low in calories you can eat a lot of them and still not gain weight.

The carbs in vegetables are easier for your body to break down and use than the carbs in things like pasta or bread. That means that your body will quickly break down the carbs in the vegetables that you eat and use those carbs for fuel instead of storing them as fat.

The vitamins and minerals in vegetables will help your body repair damaged tissue, keep muscles strong, and keep your body working the way it's supposed to. Vegetables keep your body in balance.

Try New Vegetables

One of the biggest reasons why people say they don't eat vegetables is that they find vegetables boring. But there are hundreds of vegetables that you're not eating.

Most people only try the same 9-10 vegetables they have been eating since they were children.

In order to make vegetables more appealing try some different types of vegetables.

Eating seasonally is a fabulous way to try different kinds of vegetables as well as save money because seasonal vegetables are always cheaper than vegetables that have to be shipped in from other places.

Visit a local farmer's market and check out the many different kinds of seasonal vegetables available. You can also join a farm share program where you pay a fee and the farm delivers farm fresh seasonal vegetables to your door.

Here are a few easy ways to get more vegetables into your daily diet:

- Swap vegetables for pasta and rice with dinner.

- Eat a different kind of salad every day for lunch.

- Serve vegetables and healthy dip as an appetizer.

- Keep a container of cut up vegetables at work for a quick snack.

- Throw some spinach into your morning omelet.

- Make a vegetable soup.

Eating Habit #4 – Drink More Water

How much water do you drink each day?

Chances are it's not enough. Studies have shown that people underestimate how much water they should be drinking each day.

The body is 70% water and unless you are replenishing the fluids the body loses each day you won't be healthy. Drinking water also is essential if you want to lose weight.

Water and Weight Loss

Water is critically important when it comes to weight loss and fat loss.

Drinking water will help flush out all the toxins from your cells which will keep your body healthy. Drinking water will also make you feel full which will lead to eating less and eventually weight loss.

Drinking a glass of water before each meal will make you feel full faster so that you don't want to eat as much. Drinking water instead of having an afternoon snack will make you feel full without eating a high calorie snack.

Drinking water will also help your muscles stay strong, and the more muscle you have the more calories you will burn.

Water and the Brain

Drinking water is essential for healthy brain function. When you are dehydrated you will find it hard to focus and you may be sleepy.

When that happens your brain will tell your body to have a snack in order to wake up and get through the day. That's when you will reach for sugary carb-laden snacks and drinks that will give you a boost of energy. But water is the best booster in the world.

Instead of reaching for a candy bar when you're tired or can't focus on work, reach for a bottle of water instead.

Water infused with vegetables or fruit will give you a quick jump start so that you will have the energy to get through your day, go workout, and take care of all your responsibilities.

The biggest reason why people don't drink enough water is that they think it's not convenient. But it's easy to keep water with you all day, if you just get creative and invest in a few simple tools. Use these tips to drink more water every day:

- Keep a pitcher of water in the fridge so it's ice cold and ready to go all the time.

- Put some cucumber slices, lemon wedges, or berries into an infusion pitcher to make tasty flavored water.

- Buy a water bottle and carry it with you wherever you go.

- Drink a glass of water or tea before every meal.

Eating Habit #5 - Cut Down On Caffeine

One of the things causing you to have excess belly fat could be your daily caffeine consumption. High calorie coffee drinks contain a lot more calories than most people think.

A large coffee drink can have 1000 calories or more. But it's not just high calorie fancy coffee drinks that can cause belly fat.

Most people think that caffeine will help them lose weight because it is a stimulant but that's not the case. Coffee or foods that are high in caffeine can actually cause you to gain belly fat. And that belly fat can be extremely hard to get rid of because it's caused by a hormone, called Cortisol.

Cortisol and Belly Fat

Cortisol is a hormone that your body pumps out when you are under a lot of stress. Not getting enough sleep can trigger Cortisol production in the body. So can stress at work or dealing with a lot of stress at home. But caffeine also causes the body to produce Cortisol because it stimulates the brain and nervous system.

If you drink too much caffeine your body has a "fight or flight" response the same way it would if you were in a life or death situation.

The body starts pumping out adrenaline and Cortisol.

When there's too much Cortisol in your body, the body will hang onto fat and store it, usually around your belly, in case you need to burn it for energy later. But when you don't use it for energy it just stays around your midsection. And every time you have too much caffeine your belly gets bigger and bigger thanks to Cortisol.

Cutting Caffeine

That doesn't mean that you need to give up your daily morning coffee though.

Just cutting down on the amount of caffeine that you consume each day is enough to lower the Cortisol levels in your body.

If you need your morning cup of coffee have just one cup, then switch to a lower caffeine drink like decaf coffee or tea.

Don't drink caffeine after noon. Don't drink sodas either because many sodas have more caffeine than a cup of coffee. There are other ways that you can lower your Cortisol levels too, which help you lose belly fat.

These activities can help lower your Cortisol levels:

- Yoga

- Meditation

- Walking

- Gentle Exercise

- Napping

Eating Habit #6 - Snack Smart

You'd be surprised how many calories you can rack up each day snacking.

Snacking is one of the most common reasons why people gain weight, especially around the midsection.

If you work at a job where you are sitting all day and you spend a lot of the day snacking those extra calories can add up to excess belly fat in a very short amount of time.

Eating frequently throughout the day can be good for weight loss, but only if you eat the right things.

Six Small Meals a Day

One of the best ways to lose weight is to eat six small meals each day instead of three large meals.

Ideally you should eat a snack size meal every few hours. But that doesn't mean you should be popping open a bag of chips every couple hours or eating candy bars.

What you should be eating are protein heavy snacks like cheese or eggs with some vegetables and maybe some fruit.

Healthy snacking can be a major fat buster because it turns your body into fat burning machine.

Protein Power

When you eat primarily protein you will burn fat faster for several reasons.

One of those reasons is that protein rebuilds muscle, and the more muscle you have the more calories you burn. Even when you are just sitting you will burn more calories if you have more muscle.

Protein also makes you feel full so that you don't eat as much. A small protein rich snack will keep you full for hours, but a carb heavy snack will make you feel hungry again quickly and all those carbs will end up stored in your body as fat.

The secret to eating healthy protein snacks instead of carb heavy snacks is preparation. You may not be able to go cook a burger when you want a snack but you can bring a couple of hardboiled eggs with you to work, to the gym, or anywhere else you go.

Protein bars are convenient and can stay in a desk drawer or a purse indefinitely.

Here are some other easy ways to keep protein snacks handy:

- Beef jerky is pure protein and easy to store.

- Make a salad in a jar and store it in the office refrigerator for a quick and healthy snack.

- Cook some eggs, cheese and spinach in a muffin tin so that you have small snack size frittatas and keep them in the freezer. Microwave a couple for a quick protein snack.

Eating Habit #7 – Swap Foods

Food swaps are a great way to change the way that you eat without sacrificing the foods that you love.

If you avoid dieting because you don't want to have to deprive yourself of things you really like to eat you can use simple swaps to make those foods healthier.

When you swap out some of the worst ingredients in the dishes you love you can cut calories, carbs, and unhealthy sugar, which will help you burn that belly fat and feel better.

Why Food Swapping Works So Well

Food swaps are one of the easiest ways to change your diet because in most dishes you can't even tell that one food was swapped for another.

In some dishes the food that is swapped is even more delicious than the original ingredient in the dish. Food swaps also mean that you and your family can all eat the same dishes you already enjoy. You don't have to make two separate meals at every meal just so that you can lose weight. Everyone can eat the same dish and enjoy the same healthy food.

Food swaps make it easier to eat healthy. Your family may not even realize that some of their favorite dishes contain food swaps.

Use these easy food swaps in your favorite dishes to dial up the protein, dial down the carbs, and burn belly fat:

- Swap Greek yogurt for sour cream: Greek yogurt is low in calories and packed with healthy protein.

- Swap Zoodles for Pasta Noodles: Zoodles, or noodles made from zucchini, are very trendy right now. They're also super healthy. Zoodles are low in calories and contain natural healthy carbs instead of carbs from starchy refined flour that you will find in pasta noodles. You can cut zoodles yourself or buy an inexpensive noodle maker that will make them for you.

- Swap cheese for bread: Instead of using bread to make a deli meat sandwich, use sliced cheese. Put a little mayonnaise on a slice of cheese, layer on some deli meat and top it with a slice of cheese for a snack of pure protein that will zap belly fat and keep you full.

- Swap nuts for chips: When you just have to have to a crunchy snack, eat some healthy nuts like peanuts or cashews instead of chips. Nuts can be high in calories like chips but at least they are packed with protein instead of empty calories. Cashews are also very good for your teeth.

- Eat vegetables instead of candy: Splurge and buy a tray full of fresh cut veggies to eat with a Greek yogurt dip. You'd spend just as much on candy or ice cream and the vegetables are much healthier.

Spend money on healthy foods and snacks instead of on junk food.

Eating Habit #8 - Skip Dessert

This habit can be tough, especially if you love dessert. But getting in the habit of skipping dessert can help you lose fat and maintain a healthy weight.

Dessert doesn't have to be something you eat every day. In fact, dessert is better when it's something you don't have all the time.

Desserts are often high in fat, sugar, calories and carbs so eating dessert all the time really packs on the pounds.

Often people think it's fine to treat themselves to dessert, but why treat yourself with food?

Food is fuel for your body. Look for other things to reward yourself with.

Dessert is a Once in a While Food

That doesn't mean you have to skip your favorite holiday dessert or not have birthday cake on your birthday. But it does mean that on a day-to-day basis you should just skip it.

Don't keep sweets in the house and don't prepare dessert as a part of dinner.

If you want a snack a few hours after dinner, have some vegetables with hummus or some nuts or even a piece of fruit.

The natural sugar in fruit is much easier for your body to break down than refined sugar.

You don't have to go hungry. You just have to make different food choices. Before long you won't even miss dessert.

Treats Don't Have to be Food

Instead of treating yourself to dessert every day put aside the money that you would spend on dessert and once a week buy yourself a book, or take a class, or go see a movie.

Try a yoga class or buy some hobby materials.

Stop rewarding yourself with food. You will get a lot more value out of doing something for yourself that doesn't involve food.

Buy a new journal or a new CD. Invest in yourself by learning a new skill or having some fun that isn't associated with food. You will feel better, have more fun, and you never know what new sport or hobby you might find that you enjoy.

Start by cutting out dessert just two nights each week and slowly work up to giving up dessert altogether.

Here are some fun things you can try with the money you save on dessert:

- Buy a new bike and go on a bike ride with your kids.

- Buy a pair of cozy slippers.

- Buy a water bottle so that you will start drinking more water.

- Visit a local farmer's market and buy some fresh local produce.

- Buy some gardening books and learn to grow your own vegetables.

- Take your partner to the movies.

Eating Habit #9 - Cut Out Refined Sugar

Refined sugar is something that has been proven to cause belly fat. That's because refined sugar is a simple carbohydrate.

Complex carbohydrates are the carbs that give you energy. Simple carbs are just empty calories that end up as fat in the body because they have no nutritional value.

Most people don't even realize how much refined sugar they are eating every day because they don't realize that nearly every prepared food or restaurant food contains at least some refined sugar and some foods contain huge amounts of it.

Hidden in Plain Sight

If you think that just because you don't put refined sugar in your coffee or eat sugary snacks you're safe from refined sugar you're wrong.

Every day foods that you wouldn't think contain sugar actually do have sugar in them. Things like spaghetti sauce, salad dressing, canned vegetables, yogurt, crackers, breads and other foods.

Over the years food manufacturers started adding more and more sugar to their products so that people would buy them. Prepared foods like boxed mashed potatoes, stuffing and other foods also have hidden sugar in them. Most people are eating 3x the amount of sugar they should be eating daily without even realizing it.

How to Cut Your Sugar Consumption

First you need to stop drinking soda, fruit juice with added sugar, and fancy coffee drinks that are packed with sugar.

Smoothies also contain added sugar, even though they are supposed to be healthy.

The next thing you need to do is start-preparing food from scratch.

It may seem daunting but it's really not as hard as you think.

Preparing your own food from raw ingredients will ensure that you are not eating a lot of sugar that you don't want to be eating. Also start reading food labels closely to find out if they have hidden sugar.

If you aren't feeling secure enough to start cooking from scratch then look for diabetic friendly foods when you shop.

Diabetic foods will have lower sugar content and no added sugar.

Other ways you can cut your intake of refined sugar include:

- Switch to a natural sugar substitute. Use that for coffee, baking, or cereal.

- Use natural, locally grown honey as a sweetener. Honey has a wide range of health benefits.

- Drink water instead of bottled tea and soda.

- Look for dark chocolate bars, which have lower sugar content.

- Eat more fruit and naturally sweet foods.

- Make your own sauces and dips.

- Buy unsweetened plain yogurt and flavor it yourself with berries and spices.

Eating Habit #10 - Eat More Fat

That sounds crazy right?

For years people have been told that low fat diets are the only healthy diets and that eating fat makes you fat. But that's not the case.

In fact, not eating any fat just makes you hungry and it actually makes it harder for your body to burn fat. The body needs fat in order to function.

However, that doesn't mean you can go out and start eating cupcakes all day long. You need to eat healthy fats in order to lose fat.

When you eat healthy fats you will feel full longer and you won't eat as much. Your body will also function better and burn more fat for energy, which will help you lose fat.

Healthy Fat Vs. Unhealthy Fat

There really are healthy fats that you should be eating, even though that might sound too good to be true.

The fats in foods like yogurt, avocadoes, nuts, seeds and oils like olive oil are healthy and you should be eating more of them. About ten percent of your daily calories should come from healthy fats if you want to lose weight.

Diets like the Mediterranean diet, which are high in protein and healthy fats, are strongly recommended by doctors because they provide the protein and fat that many people are lacking in their daily diets. Even the fat in some meat like bacon can be healthy if you don't overdo it.

Low Fat Is Making You Fat

Low fat diet food is something that you should avoid.

Foods that are advertised as low fat really just use chemical sweeteners and other additives to make the food taste good while removing things like cream and butter, which are healthy fats.

Those chemical additives contribute directly to weight gain and belly fat.

It's much better to eat foods with natural fat in them than to eat supposed low fat food if you want to burn belly fat.

So stop denying yourself healthy food that contains fat. Those foods usually contain high amounts of protein as well as healthy fat.

Here are some of the natural healthy fats you should be eating more of:

- Fish

- Nuts

- Olive Oil

- Butter

- Eggs

- Avocados

- Nut Butters like Peanut Butter or Almond Butter

Did You Enjoy The Exercise Less System?

Buy this book TODAY at:

TopFitnessAdvice.com/go/books

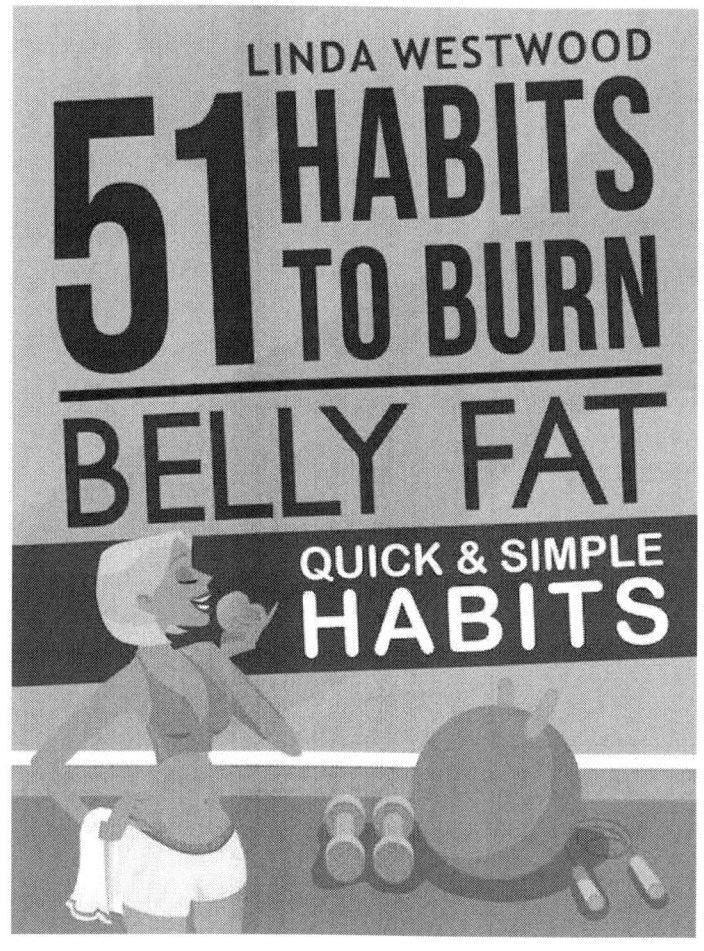

Disclaimer

This book and related sites provide wellness management information in an informative and educational manner only, with information that is general in nature and that is not specific to you, the reader. The contents of this site are intended to assist you and other readers in your personal wellness efforts. Consult your physician regarding the applicability of any information provided in our sites to you.

Nothing in this book should be construed as personal advices or diagnosis, and must not be used in this manner. The information provided about conditions is general in nature. This information does not cover all possible uses, actions, precautions, side-effects, or interactions of medicines, or medical procedures. The information in this site should not be considered as complete and does not cover all diseases, ailments, physical conditions, or their treatment.

You should **consult with your physician before beginning any exercise, weight loss, or healthcare program**. This book **should not** be used in place of a call or visit to a competent health-care professional. You should consult a health care professional before adopting any of the suggestions in this book or before drawing inferences from it.

Any decision regarding treatment and medication for your condition should be made with the advice and consultation of a qualified health care professional. If you have, or suspect you have, a health-care problem, then you should immediately contact a qualified health care professional for treatment.

No Warranties: The authors and publishers don't guarantee or warrant the quality, accuracy, completeness, timeliness, appropriateness or suitability of the information in this book, or of any product or services referenced by this site.

The information in this site is provided on an "as is" basis and the authors and publishers make no representations or warranties of any kind with respect to this information. This site may contain inaccuracies, typographical errors, or other errors.

Liability Disclaimer: The publishers, authors, and other parties involved in the creation, production, provision of information, or delivery of this site specifically disclaim any responsibility, and shall not be held liable for any damages, claims, injuries, losses, liabilities, costs, or obligations including any direct, indirect, special, incidental, or consequences damages (collectively known as "Damages") whatsoever and howsoever caused, arising out of, or in connection with the use or misuse of the site and the information contained within it, whether such Damages arise in contract, tort, negligence, equity, statute law, or by way of other legal theory.

Made in the USA
Lexington, KY
10 November 2016